# Atlas of Neonatal Electroencephalography

Third Edition

# Atlas of Neonatal Electroencephalography

## Third Edition

**Eli M. Mizrahi**, M.D.
*Head, Peter Kellaway Section of Neurophysiology*
*Vice Chairman, Department of Neurology*
*Professor of Neurology and Pediatrics*
*Baylor College of Medicine*
*Chief, Neurophysiology Service*
*The Methodist Hospital and Texas Children's Hospital*
*Houston, Texas*

**Richard A. Hrachovy**, M.D.
*Professor of Neurology*
*Peter Kellaway Section of Neurophysiology*
*Baylor College of Medicine*
*Director, Neurophysiology Services*
*Director, Epilepsy Center*
*Veteran's Administration Medical Center*
*Attending, Neurophysiology Service*
*The Methodist Hospital and Texas Children's Hospital*
*Houston, Texas*

**Peter Kellaway**, PH.D.
*Professor of Neurology and Neuroscience*
*Founder, Section of Neurophysiology*
*Baylor College of Medicine*
*Senior Attending, Neurophysiology Service*
*The Methodist Hospital and Texas Children's Hospital*
*Houston, Texas*

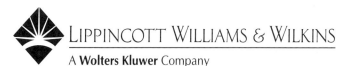

LIPPINCOTT WILLIAMS & WILKINS
A **Wolters Kluwer** Company

Philadelphia · Baltimore · New York · London
Buenos Aires · Hong Kong · Sydney · Tokyo

*Acquisitions Editor: Anne M. Sydor*
*Developmental Editor: Grace Caputo*
*Production Editor: Robin E. Cook*
*Manufacturing Manager: Colin Warnock*
*Cover Designer: Christine Jenny*
*Compositor: Maryland Composition*
*Printer: Edwards Brothers*

© 2004 by LIPPINCOTT WILLIAMS & WILKINS
530 Walnut St.
Philadelphia, PA 19106 USA
LWW.com

Printed in the USA

**Library of Congress Cataloging-in-Publication Data**

Mizrahi, Eli M.
    Atlas of neonatal electroencephalography.—3rd ed./Eli M. Mizrahi, Richard A. Hrachovy, Peter Kellaway.
      p. ; cm.
    Rev. ed. of: Atlas of neonatal electroencephalography/Janet E. Stockard-Pope, Sarah S. Werner,
Reginald G. Bickford. 2nd ed. c1992.
    Includes bibliographical references and index.
    ISBN 0-7817-3445-2
    1. Infants (Newborn)—Diseases—Diagnosis—Atlases. 2.
Electroencephalography—Atlases. 3. Pediatric neurology—Atlases. I. Hrachovy, Richard A., 1948- II.
Kellaway, Peter, 1920- III. Stockard-Pope, Janet E. Atlas of neonatal electroencephalography. IV. Title.
    [DNLM: 1. Electroencephalography—Infant, Newborn—Atlases. 2. Infant, Newborn, Diseases—
diagnosis—Atlases. 3. Neurologic Examination—Infant, Newborn—Atlases. WL 17 M685a 2003]
    RJ290.5.M59 2003
    618.92′8047547—dc21
                                               2003054340

10 9 8 7 6 5 4 3 2 1

# Contents

# Preface

The practice of neonatal electroencephalography combines clinical medicine and biomedical technology. It is based on the understanding of both the general principles of electroencephalography (EEG) interpretation and aspects unique to the neonatal period, but it is limited by a gap in our knowledge between well-characterized features of some neonatal EEG findings and those that have yet to be clearly defined by clinical investigations. In considering these factors, we have written *Atlas of Neonatal Electroencephalography* to be a single-source reference concerning neonatal EEG based on available information. Through the text, tables, and the samples of EEG recordings, we have tried to present a comprehensive view of the clinical practice of neonatal EEG for neurologists and clinical neurophysiologists, for trainees in neurology and clinical neurophysiology, and for electroneurodiagnostic technologists.

This atlas consists of chapters concerning the approach to visual analysis, artifacts of noncerebral origin, age-dependent normal findings, patterns of uncertain diagnostic significance, abnormal EEG findings, and seizures. Chapters consist of explanatory text, tables, a list of figures, and the samples themselves with their legends. We have presented information based on the available referenced literature from a diverse group of clinical investigators. However, in considering the aspects of neonatal EEG for which no studies are available and for which unresolved controversies persist, we have provided our own opinions. These have been formulated within our group, based on our collective experience, which spans more than 50 years. In addition, over the years, we have written a number of articles and reviews on neonatal electroencephalography, and we have also drawn from these works (Hrachovy, 2000; Kellaway and Hrachovy, 1981; Mizrahi, 1986; Hrachovy et al, 1990; Mizrahi and Kellaway, 1998).

This atlas has been produced at a time when many laboratories are replacing analog recording devices with digital instrumentation. Thus, we have presented a mixture of EEG samples derived from pen-and-ink and from digital, computer-based recordings. All of our samples are shown as they were recorded in the course of clinical practice in our laboratory or at the bedside in the neonatal intensive care unit without modification. Unless otherwise indicated in figure legends, the recording parameters for all EEG channels on all samples are sensitivity, 7 μV/mm; high-frequency filter, 70 Hz; low-frequency filter, 0.5 Hz; 60 Hz filter on; paper speed 30 mm/sec (analog recordings) and 10 sec/screen (digital recordings). In addition, because bedside EEG-video monitoring is becoming more available for neonates, we have provided technical information concerning this method of monitoring.

In presenting samples, we have emphasized specific components of the neonatal EEG. Our hope is that the *Atlas of Neonatals Electroencephalography* will allow the neurophysiologist to be able to recognize within a clinical recording the individual elements we have presented so as to determine their significance.

The neurophysiologist should understand the age-dependent characteristics of the neonatal EEG as well as the potential factors that may effect the developing central nervous system. Thus, throughout we have emphasized the age-dependent nature of both normal and abnormal findings of the neonatal EEG and the need to correlate them with clinical data. The most valuable report of the findings of a neonatal EEG is one with clinical relevance—a report that attempts to answer the clinical questions raised by the referring physician.

*Eli M. Mizrahi, M.D.*
*Richard A. Hrachovy, M.D.*
*Peter Kellaway, Ph.D.*
*Houston, Texas*
*April 2003*

# In Memoriam

Two months after this edition of *Atlas of Neonatal Electroencephalography* was completed, on June 25, 2003, our colleague, mentor, and friend Peter Kellaway, Ph.D., died. He was 82 years old and had maintained an active work schedule of teaching, research, and EEG interpretations up to the time of his death. He had been integrally involved in all aspects of the preparation of this atlas and worked hard to see its completion. While it might be considered the culmination of his lifelong work in the neurophysiology of the developing brain, this atlas should be thought of more as a continuation of this work, since as he often noted there is still much to learn about neonatal EEG. Dr. Kellaway was instrumental in the establishment of the electroencephalogram as an important clinical tool for diagnosis and management of neonatal cerebral disturbances and for studying the immature central nervous system in health and disease. He was an insightful, talented and generous teacher. His hope was that this atlas would stimulate others to maintain and further standards of practice and to establish new areas of research that would advance this field. His academic publication career spanned six decades—his first scientific paper appeared in 1943 and this atlas, appearing in 2003, is his last. We are honored to have had the opportunity to collaborate with him for more than twenty years and, in particular, to have worked with him on this project.

*Eli M. Mizrahi, M.D.*
*Richard A. Hrachovy, M.D.*

# Acknowledgments

We have been fortunate to collaborate with a number of valued colleagues at Baylor College of Medicine (BCM), The Methodist Hospital (TMH), and Texas Children's Hospital (TCH) in the development of our clinical and research programs in neurophysiology of the newborn. We are indebted to our colleagues in the Peter Kellaway Section of Neurophysiology, Department of Neurology, BCM, including James D. Frost, Jr., M.D., Professor of Neurology and Neuroscience; Daniel G. Glaze, M.D., Associate Professor of Pediatrics and Neurology; Merrill S. Wise, M.D., Assistant Professor of Pediatrics and Neurology; and James Crawley, M.D., Professor of Neurology (deceased, 1984),

We also are grateful to our group of electroneurodiagnostic technologists with expertise in neonatal recordings, including Nina Kagawa, R.EEG.T., Supervisor, Department of Neurophysiology, TMH (retired, 1995); Anita L. Thompson, R.EEG.T., Technical Supervisor, Department of Neurophysiology, TCH; Kelvin L. Dillard, R.EEG.T., Senior Technologist, Department of Neurophysiology, TCH; and Lisa B. Rhodes, R.EEG.T. R.EP.T., Lead Technologist, Clinical Research Center for Neonatal Seizures, TMH/BCM. The electroneurodiagnostic technologists of TCH provide EEG services to neonates 24 hours per day, 7 days per week. We appreciate their dedication, patience, and expertise in generating the technically excellent recordings that form the basis of this atlas. We also acknowledge the expert editorial assistance given to us by Katie Pierson, Senior Administrative Coordinator, Section of Neurophysiology, BCM.

We gratefully acknowledge the National Institute of Neurological Disorders and Stroke, National Institutes of Health, which has supported the Clinical Research Center for Neonatal Seizures (NS-1-12316; E.M.M., P.I.) and the Epilepsy Research Center (NS-1-1535; P.K., P.I.). In addition, research in the Section of Neurophysiology, Department of Neurology, is supported in part by the Peter Kellaway Endowment for Research of BCM. Finally, we are indebted to The Methodist Hospital and Texas Children's Hospital for the support each institution has provided in the development of clinical neurophysiology services and research in neonatal electroencephalography.

# Atlas of Neonatal Electroencephalography

Third Edition

# CHAPTER 1

# Approach to Visual Analysis and Interpretation

The basic principles of visual analysis and interpretation of the electroencephalogram (EEG) that apply to older patients (Kellaway, 2003) also generally apply to neonates, although with some additional special considerations. For example, because of the rapid rate of cerebral development in the neonatal period, the age-dependent features of the EEG become critically important. The interpretation of the neonatal EEG requires the recognition of EEG changes from conceptional ages less than 28 weeks through 44 weeks. In addition, types of abnormalities that are age-dependent also must be identified. Further, because of the special clinical problems of neonates, it is critical to understand how specific etiologic factors may affect cerebral function and, in turn, the neonatal EEG.

Nearly 40 years ago it was pointed out that the characteristics of the EEG known to be normal and, to a lesser degree, abnormal in neonates had not been established (Kellaway and Crawley, 1964); in 2003, the situation has not changed significantly. One problem is that an assumption of normality cannot be made in a newborn with the same degree of confidence as it can in older children. This is related to the brevity of the period of life available for study and the limitations of the neurologic examination. Traditionally, in studies of neonatal EEG, infants have been considered normal if they had no abnormal neurologic signs at birth and were clinically normal at the time of discharge from hospital. Some manifestations of cerebral dysfunction may not become clinically evident until a certain level of brain maturation has been achieved. In addition, to date, systematic, long-term serial studies that correlate neonatal EEG with neurologic, psychological, and behavioral development from birth to adolescence have not been carried out. As a consequence of these limitations, the significance of certain specific features of the EEG has not been established.

Despite these limitations, the imperatives of clinical practice require a clear pre-sentation of the current knowledge of neonatal EEG. The data presented in this atlas reflect more than 50 years of our experience in the study of normal and abnormal neonates. In addition, this atlas reflects the work of other investigators (Blume and Dreyfus, 1982; Clancy, Huang, and Temple, 1993; Dreyfus-Brisac, 1957; Dreyfus-Brisac, 1959; Dreyfus-Brisac, 1962; Dreyfus-Brisac, 1964; Dreyfus-Brisac, 1968; Dreyfus-Brisac, 1970; Dreyfus-Brisac, 1978; Dreyfus-Brisac and Blanc, 1956; Dreyfus-Brisac et al., 1957; Dreyfus-Brisac et al., 1961; Dreyfus-Brisac et al., 1962; Dreyfus-Brisac and Monod, 1970; Ellingson, 1958; Ellingson, 1979; Engel and Butler, 1963; Lombroso, 1979; Lombroso, 1982; Lombroso, 1985; Monod et al., 1960; Monod and Pajot, 1965; Monod et al., 1972; Sainte-Anne-Dargassies et al., 1953; Tharp et al., 1981; Torres and Anderson, 1985; Torres and Blaw, 1968; Watanabe and Iwase, 1972; Watanabe et al., 1974). In this regard, we owe a large debt to the pioneering French group led by Dreyfus-Brisac. The group's early studies of the EEGs of premature infants were conducted in a rich institutional environment that was unique in those days. They provided the basic insights that facilitated consistent progress in the development of knowledge and rational interpretation of the EEG of the newborn.

## THE PROCESS OF VISUAL ANALYSIS

In the interpretation of the EEGs of children and adults, we believe that the only data that should be considered before visual analysis is initiated are the age and the state of consciousness of the patient (Kellaway, 2003). When interpreting EEGs of neonates, the first of these should not be considered or known, because the determination of the EEG conceptional age (CA) is a critical part of the analysis and assessment of the record. It is recognized that the determination of the state of consciousness of the neonate may be difficult to determine, but as will be shown later, it may have an impact on the eventual interpretation of the recording (see Chapter 6).

Analysis of the neonatal EEG is initially directed toward the determination of CA based on detection and the recognition of the various developmental features occurring in the record (see Chapter 4). If the EEG lacks recognized developmental features that would permit the determination of CA, then this, in itself, is evidence of significant brain dysfunction. Developmental EEG features may suggest a specific CA, but a discrepancy may exist between the clinically determined CA and the EEG-derived CA; referred to as *external dyschronism.* This may arise simply from a miscalculation of the clinically determined age, and this is the most likely if the EEG is normal in all other respects. The developmental characteristics of the EEG in deep non–rapid eye movement (REM) sleep may be more immature than those of the EEG awake and in light sleep; referred to as *internal dyschronism.* In this instance, the most immature features of the deep non-REM sleep findings reflect the age at or before which a cerebral insult may have occurred.

The final step in the process of analysis is the detection and characterization of any abnormal features. These features also may be age-dependent, are described in Chapters 5 to 7, and include characterization of background activity and focal features.

As in older children and adults, visual analysis of the EEG of newborns should be an orderly process, involving a series of logical steps that result in the *technical analysis* and on which *interpretation* is based. Then, and only then, should a correlation be made with the clinical history and findings to derive a *clinical impression.* **Figure 1-1** summarizes the steps of this intellectual process.

## THE CLINICAL IMPRESSION

The neonatal EEG can be a powerful tool when applied to specific clinical questions (**Table 1-1**). However, the usefulness of the EEG in these situations will depend on the scope and quality of the information provided by the referring physician and also on the clinical neurophysiologist's understanding of the neurologic disorders of newborn.

### What Is the Conceptional Age?
The CA-dependent features of the neonatal EEG are the character of the background activity, the presence of wake–sleep stages, specific waveforms and patterns (collectively referred to as *graphoelements*), and reactivity (see Chapter 4).

Recognition of these features allows the clinical neurophysiologist to determine the CA of an infant within a 2-week epoch. In some clinical circumstances, the CA of the infant is unknown; indeterminate; or based on inconsistent data from maternal history, infant physical examination, or prenatal head ultrasound. However, determination of an accurate EEG-derived CA may add to the understanding of ongoing clinical problems and assessment of the potential risk of future difficulties.

### Is There Evidence of Focal Brain Dysfunction?
As in older children and adults, the EEG in neonates may indicate the presence of a consistent focal brain abnormality. Findings such as persistent voltage asymmetries, focal slow activity, and recurrent and persistent sharp waves, either in isolation or in combination, may indicate focal intracranial abnormalities such as subdural fluid effusion, subarachnoid hemorrhage, intracranial hemorrhage, cystic or atrophic lesions, cortical infarction, cerebral malformation, and rarely, a space-occupying lesion.

Sharp waves may suggest brain injury that is either focal when sharp waves are persistent and unifocal, or diffuse when sharp waves are multifocal (see Chapters 5 and 6). However, focal sharp waves are rarely indicative of epileptogenicity in the newborn (see Chapter 7) (Mizrahi and Kellaway, 1998). Positive rolandic sharp (PRS) waves were initially associated with the presence of intraventricular hemorrhage (IVH) in the premature infant (Dreyfus-Brisac and Monod, 1964). Subsequently, PRS waves have been shown to be associated with periventricular leukomalacia, a condition that may be a consequence of periventricular brain injury including IVH (Clancy and Tharp, 1984; Novotny et al., 1987). Focal sharp waves that recur in a periodic fashion have been associated with herpes simplex virus encephalitis (Mizrahi and Tharp, 1982; Mikati et al., 1990). It should be noted that the significance of some types of sharp waves in the neonatal EEG is unknown and is discussed further in Chapter 5.

### Is Evidence Found of Diffuse Brain Dysfunction?
The neonatal EEG may indicate the presence and degree of diffuse brain dysfunction. Although it may provide evidence of an encephalopathy and its severity, the EEG is less likely to provide information concerning etiology. Thus, similar findings of background activity may be present in infants with hypoxic–ischemic encephalopathy, central nervous system (CNS) infections, bilateral cerebral hemorrhage or infarctions, some metabolic disturbances, and other etiologic factors that may cause diffuse CNS injury.

The characterization of abnormalities of the background activity that describe the continuum of diffuse dysfunction are, from the least to the most severe: depressed and undifferentiated, suppression-burst, and isoelectric (see Chapter 6).

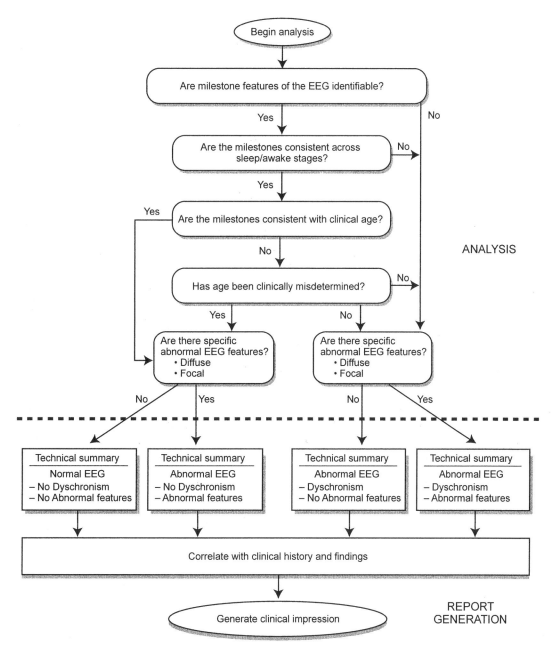

**FIG. 1–1.** Flow diagram showing the process of visual analysis and interpretation of the neonatal EEG.

**TABLE 1–1.** *Clinical questions that can be addressed by the neonatal EEG*

---

• What is the conceptional age?
• Is there evidence of focal brain dysfunction?
• Is there evidence of diffuse brain dysfunction?
• When did the brain insult occur?
• Are there clinical or electrical seizures?
• What is the neurologic prognosis?
• Is there an indication that a specific disease entity is present?

---

The timing of these findings in relation to injury may suggest both severity of the encephalopathy and its prognosis, because some abnormal findings obtained in the acute period after injury may be only transient. Additional findings that suggest diffuse brain dysfunction are those characterized by the term internal dyschronism.

### When Did the Brain Insult Occur?

No formal studies link EEG findings with the determination of the time of occurrence of diffuse brain injury. However, a number of logical assumptions have been made in the application of EEG in relation to this clinical question. As discussed earlier, internal dyschronism occurs when the developmental features of the EEG in deep non-REM sleep are more immature than those in wakefulness and light sleep and indicates that the infant has had a brain insult. The CA derived from the features in deep sleep indicates that an insult occurred at or before the developmental age associated with those specific features.

### Are Clinical or Electrical Seizures Present?

The clinical problem of neonatal seizures is discussed in Chapter 7 and in more detail elsewhere (Mizrahi and Kellaway, 1998). Recording seizures is dependent on the duration of the EEG recording and its timing. Seizures may be classified according to the temporal relation of clinical and EEG events. Electroclinical seizures are those in which clinical and EEG seizure activities overlap in time, typically with close correlation of limb, body, or facial movements to electrical discharges. Electrical-only seizures are those that occur without clinical events. Clinical-only seizures are those without any EEG correlate.

Interictal findings, such as the character of the background, may be helpful in assessing the degree and distribution of CNS dysfunction and may even suggest the degree of risk of seizure occurrence (Laroia et al., 1998). However, interictal focal sharp waves do not provide reliable markers of potential epileptogenesis. Focal sharp waves or even spikes do not always have the same implications in the neonate as they do in older children or adults and therefore may not be considered epileptiform.

### What Is the Prognosis?

Some features of the EEG that indicate focal or diffuse injury also may suggest the long-term neurologic prognosis. For example, the frequency of occurrence of PRS waves may predict the occurrence of neurologic sequelae (Blume and Dreyfus-Brisac, 1984), and a severely abnormal background activity also may suggest a poor prognosis. However, the overriding factor in the use of neonatal EEG in determination of prognosis is the evolution of findings over time in sequential studies. A single normal EEG near the time of suspected injury usually predicts a good outcome. An initial EEG with an abnormal background, even when severely abnormal, may, over time, evolve to a less abnormal or even a normal recording, depending on the nature of the brain insult. The rate of resolution, if any, will be the most predictive of outcome, rather than a single EEG at one time.

### Is an Indication of a Specific Disease Entity Present?

In general, it is unusual for the neonatal EEG to provide data that will identify specific diseases. Only a few patterns are diagnostic. PRS waves traditionally have been associated with the presence of IVH, but now are more consistently associated with periventricular leukomalacia (Clancy and Tharp, 1984). Herpes simplex virus encephalitis has been associated with the finding of periodic lateralized epileptiform discharges (Mizrahi and Tharp, 1982), although this finding also may be seen in other conditions (Hrachovy et al., 1990). The condition of holoprosencephaly is associated with a specific pattern of rapidly changing background activity (DeMyer and White, 1964). A pattern of periodic hypsarrhythmia in term infants has been associated with nonketotic hyperglycinemia and other inborn errors of metabolism (Aicardi, 1985; Ohtahara, 1978). All of these patterns are discussed in Chapter 6.

# CHAPTER 2

# Techniques of Recording the Neonatal Electroencephalogram*

## GENERAL PRINCIPLES

The general principles of recording the electroencephalogram (EEG) in older children and adults apply to the recording of the EEG in neonates, with some important additions and exceptions. Guidelines for the recording of the neonatal EEG have been established by the American Clinical Neurophysiology Society (ACNS, 1986) and the International Federation of Clinical Neurophysiology (De Weerd et al., 1999). In addition, a number of reports have detailed the technical aspects of neonatal EEG recording (Hanley, 1981; Kagawa, 1973; Mizrahi, 1986). These guidelines and reports were developed when only analog recordings were made. Technologic advances of digital recordings (Levy et al., 1998; Van Cott and Brenner, 1998) and bedside EEG-video monitoring (Kellaway, 1986; Mizrahi and Kellaway, 1987) have created the need for further delineation of their application in the neonate.

### Personnel

Critical to the recording of neonatal EEG is a well-trained staff of electroneurodiagnostic technologists (ENDTs) with expertise in the recording of newborn and young infants. Such technologists provide the expert interface between the patient and the interpreting clinical neurophysiologist by ensuring technical excellence, a clinical understanding of neonatal care, the detailed observation of normal and abnormal infant behaviors, a good working relationship with nursing staff, and an empathetic relationship with parents. The recording of a neonatal EEG is not just the recording of an EEG on a miniaturized adult or child—technologists require specialized training to produce clinically relevant records.

Clinical neurophysiologists with expertise in the interpretation of neonatal EEGs also are essential. The neurophysiologist also should have a thorough familiarity with the clinical problems that neonates may encounter to provide individualized and clinically relevant interpretations and clinical correlations.

It is essential to provide neonatal EEG services 24 hours/day, 7 days/week because the most frequent reasons for referral are suspicion of clinical seizures and acute alteration of mental status. For the EEG to be valuable in the assessment of such affected infants, it must be available around the clock. This requires the availability of specialized technologists and clinical neurophysiologists.

Biomedical engineering support staff and, more recently, computer technologists are often overlooked as essential members of the neonatal EEG team. These professionals ensure that instrumentation is well maintained, ready for use on an emergency basis, and quickly repaired if necessary.

## DATA COLLECTION

The findings of the neonatal EEG are most valuable when considered in relation to an individual patient's history and clinical findings. To ensure maximal clinical relevance, the ENDT obtains basic information about each neonate to be recorded. This information is listed in **Table 2-1** and includes standard demographic data, description of the recording environment, documentation of reason for referral, details of the medical history, a list and timing of medications, and the specifics of the infant's general medical condition. This information may be ob-

*Additional contributors to this chapter are Lisa B. Rhodes, R.EEG.T. R.EP.T., Lead Electroneurodiagnostic Technologist, Clinical Research Center for Neonatal Seizures, The Methodist Hospital; and Anita L. Thompson, R.EEG.T., Technical Supervisor, Clinical Neurophysiology Laboratories, Texas Children's Hospital, Houston, Texas.

**TABLE 2–1.** *Data collection for recording of the neonatal EEG*

I. Patient demographic information
    A. Name
    B. Date of birth (chronologic age)
    C. Stated estimated gestational age at birth
    D. Birthweight
II. Recording environment
    A. Location
        1. Hospital nursery
            a. Routine
            b. Special care units
        2. Laboratory
    B. Crib type
        1. Open bassinette
        2. Isolette
        3. Infant warmer
    C. Additional instrumentation
        1. Monitors
        2. Ventilator
        3. Phototherapy
        4. Extracorporeal membrane oxygenation
        5. Other
III. Reason for referral
    A. Altered mental status
    B. Determination of conceptional age
    C. Identification of diffuse cerebral disturbance
    D. Identification of focal cerebral lesion
    E. Suspected seizures
        1. Description of suspected clinical event
        2. Timing and duration of events
    F. Other
IV. Medical history
    A. Prenatal
        1. Maternal history
        2. Pregnancy history
    B. Perinatal
        1. Route of delivery
        2. Apgar score
        3. Requirements for delivery room resuscitation
    C. Postnatal
        1. Hospital course since delivery
        2. History at home after initial discharge

V. Medications
    A. Drug
        1. Sedation
        2. Antiepileptic drugs
        3. Paralytic agents
        4. Other
    B. Dose
    C. Timing
        1. Date
        2. Hours
        3. Routine schedule
    D. Route of administration
    E. Recipient
        1. Neonate
        2. Maternal (with potential neonatal effect)
VI. General medical condition
    A. Medical treatments
        1. Limb restraints
        2. Intravascular lines
        3. Intubation
        4. Gastric tube access
        5. Other
    B. Physical condition
        1. Body position
        2. Recent surgical wounds
        3. Healed scars
        4. Scalp swelling
        5. Ventriculoperitoneal shunt
    C. Degree of infant comfort
        1. Comfortable, without distress
        2. Irritable when handled, but consolable
        3. Inconsolable
    D. Apparent mental status
        1. Awake and alert
        2. Difficult to arouse
        3. Nonresponsive
    E. Feeding
        1. Type
        2. Route (oral, tube)
        3. Schedule
        4. Time of last feeding

tained from the infant's referring physician, parents, or hospital chart; thus the technologist must be trained to be familiar with the medical issues of neonates. To aid in data collection, well-designed data-collection forms tailored for use in each neurophysiology laboratory eventually become part of the infant's laboratory and hospital medical record.

## INFANT PREPARATION

The recording of the neonatal EEG may be routine in special care units where parents become familiar with the many medical procedures performed on their infants. However, it may be a unique experience for the infant and parents in the outpatient setting. In either circumstance, the ENDT should attempt to put the family at ease by explaining the procedure and answering any questions and concerns.

The clinical state of infants may vary: they may be content and comfortable, difficult to console, irritable, excessively sleepy or lethargic, or comatose. The technologist must consider the state of each infant and determine the best method to make the infant as comfortable as possible to obtain a complete recording. This may require having the infant fed, having diapers changed, adjusting room temperature and, often, just prolonging the recording until the infant becomes comforted. The purpose of these efforts is to facilitate a recording of spontaneous sleep cycles as well as an awake portion.

## ELECTRODE PLACEMENT

The International 10-20 System of Electrode Placement (Jasper, 1958) has been modified for recording neonates (**Fig. 2–1**) (Kellaway and Crawley, 1964). This is to accommodate the neonate's immature frontal lobes that do not extend as anteriorly relative to the skull compared with those in older children and adults. Typically, nine scalp positions are used (F1, F2, C3, C4, Cz, T3, T4, O1, O2), although others may be added. In addition, electrodes are placed at A1 and A2, and a ground electrode is placed either at mid-forehead or on a mastoid region. Because digital recordings are fundamentally referential, an additional reference electrode position may be needed (typically noncephalic), although some instruments provide a so-called "internal" reference. The F1 and F2 electrode positions are 20% of the inion–nasion distance above the nasion and 10% of the circumferential measurement from the midline. For neonates, placement of all of the standard electrodes of the International System would result in such close spacing on the infant's scalp that many electrodes would record overlapping, and thus redundant, electrical fields. The optimal number of electrodes has not been determined, but clinical

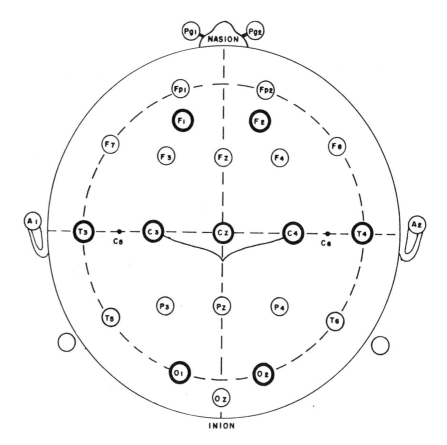

**FIG. 2–1.** Electrode placement for the neonatal electroencephalogram designated by bolded circles.

experience in our laboratories has shown that the nine cephalic positions designated are sufficient to characterize the normal neonatal EEG and to detect, localize, and characterize major abnormalities.

After head measurement, the scalp is prepared with slight abrasion at each electrode site with a mild abrasive gel, using the soft end of a cotton applicator. This may cause slight erythema at the site, but this is a temporary effect. Conductive paste is used to secure the electrodes. A ball of cotton is placed over each electrode, and the electrode array is finally secured with paper tape. Paste can be used successfully for even lengthy recordings when applied and attended to by experienced ENDTs. Collodion is typically not used for routine neonatal EEG for a number of reasons. The environment in which collodion is applied must be well ventilated because it is flammable and may be toxic to the lungs. This is a particular problem for infants in special care units who may be in confined areas such as isolettes that may concentrate fumes and for those infants with already compromised pulmonary function.

## POLYGRAPHIC PARAMETERS

Polygraphic measures are integral to the recording of the EEG to assist in characterizing sleep states, eye movements, muscle contractions, cardiac rhythms, and respiratory patterns (ACNS, 1986; DeWeerd, 1999; Hanley, 1981; Kagawa, 1973; Mizrahi, 1990). The same procedures are followed for electrode application as described earlier for scalp electrodes. The basic polygraphic recording parameters are discussed later.

### Electrooculogram
The electrooculogram (EOG) is recorded to detect and characterize eye movements. This assists in staging sleep and in the determination of the origin of some electrical potentials recorded in anterior cephalic electrodes that may have been generated by eye movement. For bipolar EOG recordings, one electrode is placed below and lateral to the outer canthus of one eye, and one, above and slightly lateral to the nasion (**Fig. 2–2**). This positioning will capture both horizontal and vertical eye movements.

### Electromyogram
The submental electromyogram (EMG) is recorded to assist in sleep staging and also to characterize some oral–lingual–pharyngeal muscle movements that also may contaminate the EEG. The EMG is recorded with electrodes placed bilaterally and symmetrically, immediately under the jaw. When movements recur in limbs, EMG may be recorded, to determine the precise relation of such movements to any change in the EEG. In addition, limb movements may be detected and characterized by triaxial accelerometry (Frost et al., 1978). This device will produce an analog signal in response to movements of the limb in any plane, compared with EMG, which identifies movement only in a specific direction according to muscle groups.

### Electrocardiogram
The electrocardiogram (EKG) is monitored to assess heart rate and rhythm. One electrode is placed over the midline chest and referenced to the right ear for a sin-

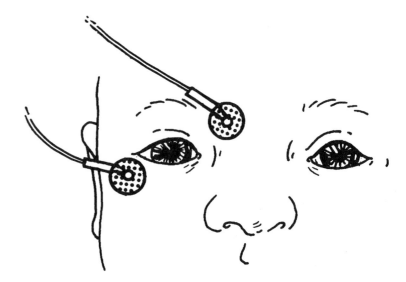

**FIG. 2–2.** Electrode placement for recording electrooculogram in the neonate.

gle-channel recording of the EKG. It also may be used to identify waveforms recorded from EEG electrodes that might have been generated by EKG.

### Respiration
Respiration is recorded to assist in sleep staging, to characterize various types of apnea, and to assist in differentiating respiratory or body movements from the EEG. The methods used for the recording of respiration may be complex. The most complete method of characterizing respiration is by measurement of abdominal movement (typically with a strain gauge or pneumograph adapted to abdominal placement), thoracic movement (with a strain gauge, bipolar electrodes, or pneumograph adapted to thoracic placement), air flow at the nares or mouth (with a thermocouple device or other flow-measurement devices), end-expiratory $CO_2$ and $O_2$ saturation with a pulse oximeter.

### Specialized Polygraphic Measures
A number of other parameters can be measured time-locked to EEG. These are most often used in research protocols or special clinical circumstances. The physiologic measure of greatest interest is systemic blood pressure. Intraarterial blood pressure can be measured from an indwelling catheter already placed for clinical

needs and, via a transducer blood pressure can be displayed numerically on a video screen or as an analog waveform on the recording.

## MONTAGE SELECTION

Major strategies in the recording of the neonatal EEG are the documentation of wake/sleep cycles, the characterization of reactivity of the record to stimulation and identification of age-dependent *graphoelements* (see Chapter 4). These are best achieved in a sustained recording by using a single, bipolar montage with broad coverage over the scalp. In the recording of older children and adults, localization of focal abnormalities often requires the use of several montages; however, because of the range of abnormalities in neonates and the overriding need to characterize state changes over time, multiple montages are not used. A typical montage, with adequate coverage over the scalp, including the required channels with a Cz electrode placement, is given in **Table 2–2**. This recommendation has been developed for analog recordings. Digital recording of the neonatal EEG provides the opportunity to examine various waveforms with different montages after recordings are complete. New data obtained from these recordings may result in additional guidelines for neonatal recordings.

**TABLE 2–2.** *Sample montage selection*

| | |
|---|---|
| Channel 1 | F1-C3 |
| Channel 2 | F2-C4 |
| Channel 3 | C3-O1 |
| Channel 4 | C4-O2 |
| Channel 5 | T3-C3 |
| Channel 6 | C3-Cz |
| Channel 7 | Cz-C4 |
| Channel 8 | C4-T4 |
| Channel 9 | F1-T3 |
| Channel 10 | F2-T4 |
| Channel 11 | T3-O1 |
| Channel 12 | T4-O2 |
| Channel 13 | EOG |
| Channel 14 | EMG |
| Channel 15 | EKG |
| Channel 16 | RESP (pneumograph) |
| Channel 17 | Time code[a] |

[a]Instrumentation dependent, if time-synchronized video is used with analog/paper recordings.

## INSTRUMENT SETTINGS

Instrument settings used at the onset of recording are listed in **Table 2–3**. The filter settings and sensitivity of the EEG channels should be the same as those for EOG to allow accurate comparison of waveforms to differentiate cerebral activity from that of ocular origin. Paper speed is set at 30 mm/sec for analog recordings or 10 sec/screen or "page" for digital recordings. These paper-speed settings are used in many laboratories in the United States and are used in this atlas. However, several laboratories, particularly those with ties to the French school of recording, use a slow speed: 15 mm/sec or 20 sec/screen or "page."

## VIDEO

Over the past several years, considerable interest has been expressed in time-synchronized video-EEG monitoring of neonates (Boylan et al., 2002; Bye et al., 1997; Mizrahi and Kellaway, 1987). These studies used these techniques in the research setting. Only recently have other centers begun to record video with EEG routinely for clinical purposes in neonates. At the outset, it may seem as if the addition of video to the recording of neonatal EEG would be relatively easy, particularly with the introduction of new, light-weight, low-light, digital video cameras added to portable digital EEGs. However, many of the difficulties that were present during the development of these techniques still persist.

### Nursery Environment

The most challenging aspect of neonatal EEG video monitoring is effective integration of recording efforts with the essential activities of the nursery. Instrumentation, camera mount, electrode cables, and junction box must all be placed not to interfere with the ongoing care of the neonate. A good working relationship between the ENDT and the nurse caring for the infant is essential for optimal recording. It also is important to keep the video image as free as possible from personnel and instruments that block the camera view. In addition, during paroxysmal clinical events, it is essential for personnel not to interfere with the recording of the entire seizure. The ambient temperature of the recording environment should be controlled as well as possible. It is important to keep the infant warm and covered. However, for infants with suspected seizures, it is essential that the infants remain uncovered, with all limbs in full view of the camera. These concerns must be addressed with nursing staff at the onset of the recording session at the bedside and with parents.

**TABLE 2–3.** *Initial instrument settings*

**EEG channels**

| | |
|---|---|
| Sensitivity[a] | 7 $\mu$V/mm |
| Time-constant[b] | 0.3 sec |
| Low-frequency filter | 0.5 Hz |
| High-frequency filter | 70 Hz |
| Notch filter (60 Hz, 50 Hz) | Off |
| Display time | |
|     Paper speed | 30 mm/sec |
|     Screen display | 10 sec/screen |

**Polygraphic channels**

| | EOG[c] | EMG[d] | RESP[d] | EKG[d] |
|---|---|---|---|---|
| Sensitivity | 7 $\mu$V/mm | 7 $\mu$V/mm | 7 $\mu$V/mm | 300 $\mu$V/mm |
| Time-constant | 0.3 sec | 0.03 sec | 0.3 sec | 0.3 sec |
| Low-frequency filter | 0.5 Hz | 5 Hz | 0.5 Hz | 0.5 Hz |
| High-frequency filter | 70 Hz | 70 Hz | 70 Hz | 70 Hz |
| Notch filter (60 Hz, 50 Hz) | Off | Off | Off | Off |

EOG, electrooculogram; EMG, electromyogram; EKG, electrocardiogram.

[a]For a digital recording, a 7 $\mu$V signal should produce a vertical deflection equivalent to 1/30 of the horizontal distance spanned by 1 second.

[b]The use of time-constant or low-frequency filter is instrumentation dependent.

[c]EOG settings remain the same as EEG settings for comparison of simultaneously recorded waveforms.

[d]EMG, RESP (pneumograph), and EKG settings may be adjusted to optimize display.

## Infant Positioning

Infants may be positioned by nursing or attending physician staff for clinical purposes. A number of constraints occur in maintaining a good video image: Limbs with intravascular line placements may be restrained; agitated infants may be swaddled; some infants may be intubated with limited range of head and neck movement; wound dressings may be present; or infants must remain covered because of temperature instability. These and other problems must be addressed to obtain the best video image for each study.

## Camera Mount

The camera mount must be stable and must not "jitter" or bounce with movement of personnel around the EEG instrument. In addition, the camera must be mounted so that it is directly above the neonate to provide a full view of all limbs and head without the distortion that comes from a camera placed at the foot or to the side of the infant.

## Lighting

Lighting in neonatal special care areas can be suboptimal for video recording. Ambient light is dictated by clinical needs and day/night cycles imposed for optimal infant adaptation. Some cameras considered "low-light" still do not provide an adequate image. When additional light is used to enhance picture quality, additional problems may arise. Added light may provide added heat and cause the infant to perspire, enhancing sweat artifact. Added light also may provide stark shadows and obscure the image of limbs. These problems must be considered before beginning video recordings and must be corrected when encountered during monitoring.

## Potential for Missed Events

A potential is always present for missing the video recording of important paroxysmal clinical events. The optimal video recordings are those time-linked with

EEG, but much can be determined from the video image alone. To maximize video-recording yield, the technologist must first arrange the video camera and begin video recording. This can start immediately after the EEG instrument is brought to the bedside or the infant is brought to the laboratory. Video recording continues through the gathering of historical data and preparation of the infant for EEG. It is terminated only after all electrodes are removed, the infant is cleaned, and the instrument is removed.

## RECORDING PROTOCOLS

The most successful and clinically relevant neonatal EEG recordings are those in which objectives and strategies are identified before the beginning of each study. Advance planning is essential. This can be based on a basic algorithm adaptable to individual recording circumstances (**Fig. 2–3**). The basic tasks are to obtain historical data, determine the reason for referral, initiate technical recordings, examine the EEG in real time, observe the infant for clinical behaviors, record the infant in sleep and wakefulness, and attempt to provoke abnormal paroxysmal clinical events.

Close observation of the patient at all times is particularly important when recording a neonatal EEG. The record should be annotated when behavioral or autonomic changes occur or when other events happen that may affect the record. It is important that the technologist and clinical neurophysiologist know what behaviors suspected by the referring physician are thought to be clinical seizures. In addition, if the type of paroxysmal behavior for which the infant was referred occurs during the recording, the event should be noted and described. Other abnormal behaviors also should be noted on the record at their time of occurrence.

Some behaviors currently thought to be seizures can be elicited by tactile stimulation and suppressed by restraint or repositioning of the infant's limbs or trunk. Therefore, bedside maneuvers to elicit or suppress such clinical behaviors are essential to an adequate recording of the neonatal EEG. During the recording, infants suspected of having seizures should be subjected to proprioceptive or tactile stimuli such as gentle pinching or tickling of the skin or repositioning of the head, trunk, or extremities. When tonic posturing or motor automatisms occur, the technologist should determine whether they can be stopped by repositioning

**FIG. 2–3. Flow diagram of the sequence of recording neonatal electroencephalogram (EEG) with video.** If video is not to be used, only those steps related specifically to video are eliminated, and the remainder are followed for EEG recording.

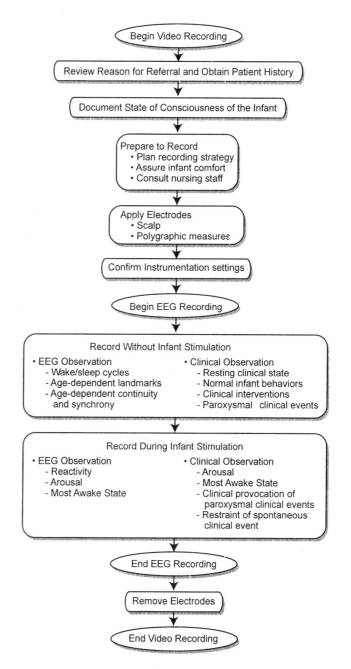

the head, trunk, or limbs. If stimulation elicits abnormal behavior, it is important to determine the relation between the intensity of the stimulus and the intensity and irradiation of the response. Whether the intensity of the behavior or the degree of irradiation can be increased by stimulating at multiple sites or by repetitive stimulation of the same site also should be determined. Finally, attempts should be made to suppress abnormal movements with light restraint.

An important concern is the duration of the neonatal EEG recording. Two considerations apply: the time it may take for the infant to experience the full cycles of sleep and wakefulness, and a sufficient period for the infant to experience clinical or electrical events. The typical minimum duration of recording for a neonatal EEG is 1 hour. A recording may be longer in an infant who may be particularly irritable and may take more time to fall asleep. Conversely, circumstances for a critically ill infant may require that the recording time be shortened. However, even a critically ill infant who is comatose and who may have an EEG that is depressed, undifferentiated, and nonreactive to stimulation may require a recording of at least a full hour because seizure discharges of the depressed brain type may eventually occur. Thus the determination of recording duration is an interactive process, based on clinical circumstances and the unfolding EEG.

# CHAPTER 3

# Artifacts

The differentiation of true brain electrical activity from extraneous artifacts is critical to the interpretation of the neonatal electroencephalogram (EEG). Traditionally, the sources of artifacts are considered in four broad categories: environment, instrumentation–patient interface, instrumentation, and physiologic potentials of noncerebral origin (Brittenham, 1990; Kellaway and Crawley, 1964; Saunders, 1979, 1985; Scher, 1985).

The identification of artifacts in a given EEG is a two-step process. The first occurs during the actual recording and is dependent on the electroneurodiagnostic technologist's (ENDT's) recognition of possible artifact sources. With this recognition, it is the ENDT's responsibility to isolate the source and resolve the problem. If this proves impossible, the ENDT will make appropriate notations on the record and on the accompanying log to characterize the activity and suggest the source. The second step of artifact identification occurs during interpretation of the EEG. Because artifacts can mimic true brain-generated waveforms (**Tables 3–1 to 3–5**), the challenge lies with the clinical neurophysiologist to make the accurate and appropriate distinctions.

## ENVIRONMENT

Although the EEG laboratory is a relatively controlled electrical environment, the neonatal intensive care unit is relatively uncontrolled. This is because of the large number of instruments used to monitor or care for infants, including phototherapy lights, ultrasound instrumentation, pumps for intravascular infusions in the umbilical and scalp vessels, and extracorporeal membrane oxygenation (ECMO) pumps (**Figs. 3–1 to 3–3**). Electrical artifacts due to external currents from these instruments may appear in all EEG channels to the same degree or may appear focally. When all of the electrode impedances are equal, the more likely the environmental current will be expressed in all channels; unequal impedances will cause the current to be expressed to a greater degree or exclusively in those channels with the highest impedance.

Additional environmental artifacts may be created or enhanced by factors such as capacitatively induced potentials from electrode wires that sway or electrostatic potentials resulting from movement of personnel around the recording area. Malfunctions and/or improper operation of equipment such as monitors connected to the patient also can result in artifactual signal induced into the EEG machine.

New ventilators recently introduced to neonatal care allow a very fast rate of respiration, and these may induce relatively high frequency electrical artifacts. Thus rate alone cannot be used to exclude potentials suspected of being generated by a ventilator.

Radio transmitters, including those used by dispatch personnel or cellular telephones, can sometimes produce artifactual signals in the EEG tracing, especially if these devices are operated within a few feet of the patient.

## RECORDING INSTRUMENTATION–PATIENT INTERFACE

The interface between the recording instrument and the patient is at the electrode site. Inadequate or unstable contact between the electrode surface and the skin may result in a sudden change in the junction potential and/or impedance that can produce extraneous potentials in affected channels. These may appear as single or repetitive rapid, spike-like waves with an abrupt upward initial phase (the so-

**TABLE 3–1.** *Sources of artifacts that can mimic EEG focal asymmetries*

Instrument–patient interface
  ○ Asymmetric electrode placement
Instrumentation
  ○ Settings (analog and digital)
  ○ Pen damping (analog only)
Physiological
  ○ Asymmetric scalp edema
  ○ Skull defects

**TABLE 3–2.** *Sources of artifacts that can mimic focal slow activity that is either random or rhythmic*

Instrument–patient interface
  ○ Inadequate electrode contact
  ○ Head positioning
  ○ Spontaneous or passive body, limb or head movements
  ○ Pulse
  ○ Respiration
Physiological
  ○ Endogenous electrical potentials
    ❑ Tongue movements
    ❑ Eye movements

**TABLE 3–3.** *Sources of artifacts that can mimic sharp waves or spikes that are either random or rhythmic*

Instrument–patient interface
  ○ Inadequate electrode contact ("pop")
  ○ Spontaneous or passive movements
    ❑ Sucking, burping, hiccupping
Instrumentation
  ○ Loosely adjusted pens (analog)
Physiological
  ○ Electrocardiogram
  ○ Electrooculogram
  ○ Facial electromyogram
Environment
  ○ Infusion pumps
  ○ Ventilator
  ○ Extracorporeal membrane oxygenation pump
  ○ Radio transmitters

**TABLE 3–4.** *Sources of artifacts that can mimic generalized activity that is either paroxysmal or sustained*

Instrumentation–patient interface
  ○ Spontaneous and passive movements
    ❑ Rocking, patting
Instrumentation
  ○ Swaying of electrode leads
Physiologic
  ○ Sweating
Environment
  ○ 60-Hz interference from adjacent instruments

called electrode "pop") (**Figs. 3–4 and 3–5**). In addition, asymmetry of the site of placement of homologous electrodes may result in significant voltage asymmetries in the EEG.

The electrode interface also may be altered by the degree to which the infant may perspire. Diffuse sweating may result in long-duration potentials that initially appear as generalized or regional slow activity (**Figs. 3–6 and 3–7**). Very slow potentials may occur because of changes caused by alterations in surface electrolyte compositions—these potentials are similar to the galvanic skin response.

Movement of the head against the bed due to respirations or other body movements may produce sharp and/or slow potentials arising from that particular electrode (**Figs. 3–8 and 3–9**). Pulse also may cause a recorded artifact by production of movement in a region adjacent to an electrode site. The head also may be moved by mechanical devices such as a ventilator or ECMO pump (**Figs. 3–10 and 3–11**). This is owing to a mechanical, or ballistic, movement induced by the instrument—a cause of artifact from these devices different from electrical interference described earlier.

Other body movements also may alter the patient–electrode interface and result in artifacts. These include limb movements that may be random, purposeful, or associated with clinical seizures and other limb or body movements (**Figs. 3–12 to**

**TABLE 3–5.** *Sources of artifact that can mimic generalized voltage depression*

Instrumentation
  ○ Instrumentation settings
Physiological
  ○ Diffuse scalp edema

**3–15**). In addition to the movements that may be caused by the infant, the infant may be moved or manipulated during comforting, feeding, medical procedures, and in the course of treatments (**Figs. 3–16 to 3–18**). Movements created to comfort the infant, such as rocking and patting the infant, may be particularly troublesome.

## RECORDING INSTRUMENTATION

The recording instrument itself can be a source of artifacts. These may be the result of malfunction at any recording level. Analog-type EEG instruments may be subject to pen misalignment and excessive damping. Digital recordings may have problems relating to malfunction of the operating system. The potential for human error also occurs in the use of either recording device. Settings for EEG channels may not be uniform, electrodes may not be correctly plugged in, and montages may not be accurately selected.

## NONCEREBRAL PHYSIOLOGIC POTENTIALS

### Alterations in Electrical Properties of Scalp or Skull

Differences may be found in impedance and volume-conduction properties over various regions of the scalp because of scalp edema. The edema may be the result of transit through the birth canal, more significant birth or other trauma, placement of intravenous lines with or without extravasation of fluid, the placement of a ventriculoperitoneal shunt, or the presence of a surgical wound. Diffuse edema may lead to a pattern of background activity that is low in amplitude in all regions. Regional or asymmetric edema may lead to a pattern of focal depression, suggesting a focal lesion if the edema is not noted. Conductive properties may be altered because of the absence of underlying skull, typically (although rarely) in the case of cranial surgery. A skull defect creates a preferential pathway for electrical current, resulting in an increased amplitude of EEG activity over the affected region.

### Vital Signs Monitoring

Heart rate and respirations are important sources of artifact on EEG. The electrocardiogram (EKG) in an infant may appear as a contaminant in one, some, or all of the EEG channels (**Figs. 3–19 and 3–20**). It may be constant or intermittent. Respirations also may appear as artifacts, whether they are spontaneous or driven by a ventilator. These artifacts may be unilateral or bilateral, depending on body and head position.

### Movements

Some movements by the infant can produce a number of endogenous electrical potentials that can be reflected in EEG channels. These movements include oral–buccal–lingual movements, such as sucking and tongue thrusting (i.e., glossopharyngeal potential); paroxysmal pharyngeal movements, such as hiccupping, burping [i.e., pharyngeal muscles and diaphragmatic electromyogram (EMG)], and jaw tremor (**Figs. 3–21 to 3–27**); ocular movements, such as eye deviations, blinking, and repetitive eye opening and closure [i.e., electrooculogram (EOG)] (**Figs. 3–28 to 3–31**); and chewing or other facial movements (i.e., temporalis, frontalis, or other facial muscle EMG) (**Figs. 3–32 to 3–37**).

## LIST OF FIGURES

### Environmental Interference

### Alternations of Electrode Impedance

### Induced by Movements

### Endogenous Noncerebral Potentials

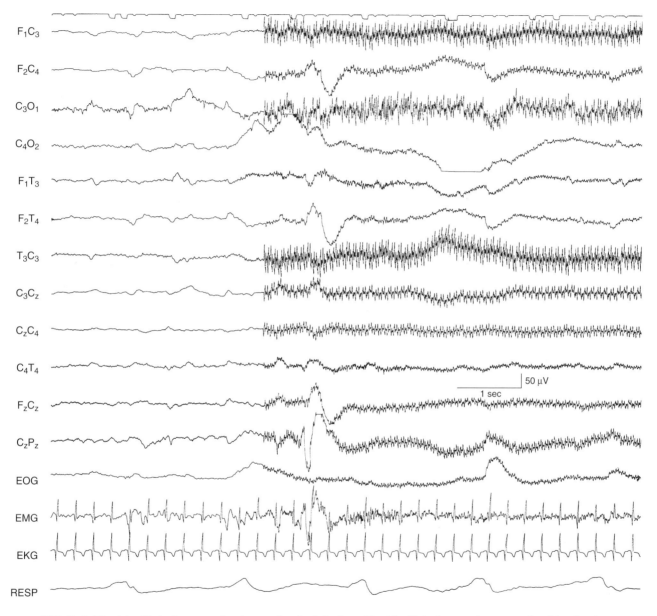

**FIG. 3–1. Electrical interference due to mechanical device.** Electrical interference is present in all leads when an infusion pump for intravenous fluids is activated at the bedside. The interference is modified in this instance by the use of a 60-Hz filter. The EEG background activity is depressed and undifferentiated in this term infant.

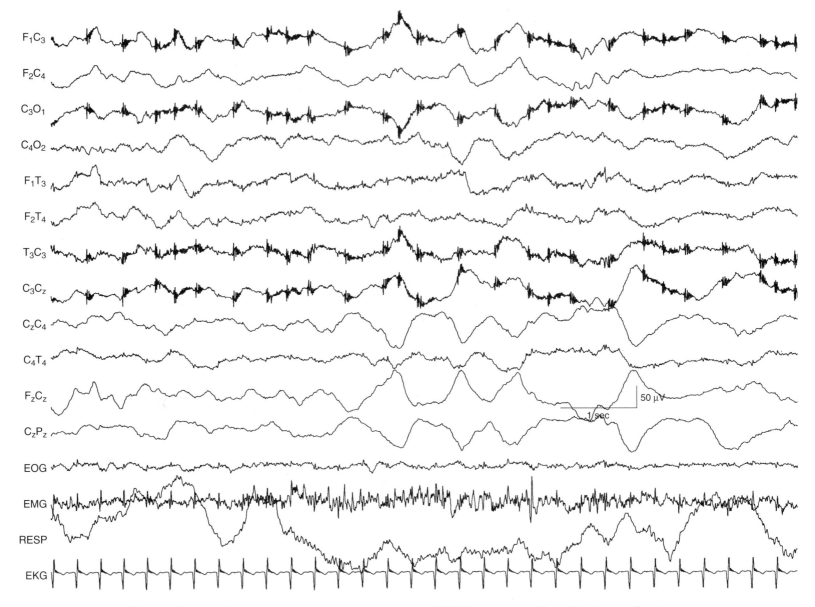

**FIG. 3–2. Electrical interference due to intensive care unit (ICU) instrumentation.** Electrical artifact is present in channels involving the C3 electrode, which has relatively high impedance compared with others. This 40-week CA infant was cared for in an ICU with monitors, ventilator, and infusion pump. The background EEG activity is undifferentiated.

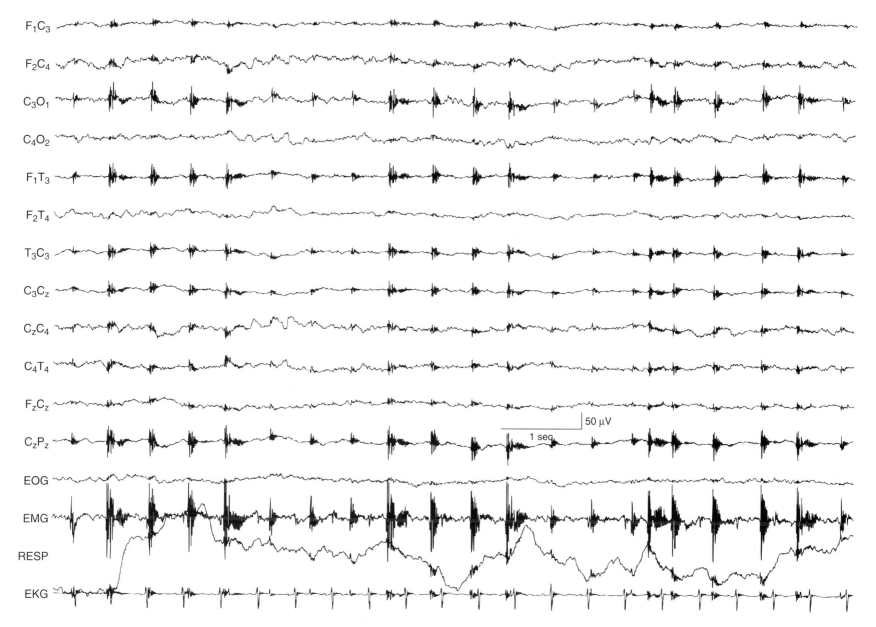

**FIG. 3–3. Periodic electrical interference due to mechanical device.** Periodic bursts of electrical interference are due to an extracorporeal membrane oxygenation pump used to support this term infant, whose background EEG is depressed and undifferentiated. The bursts correlate with rotations of the pump.

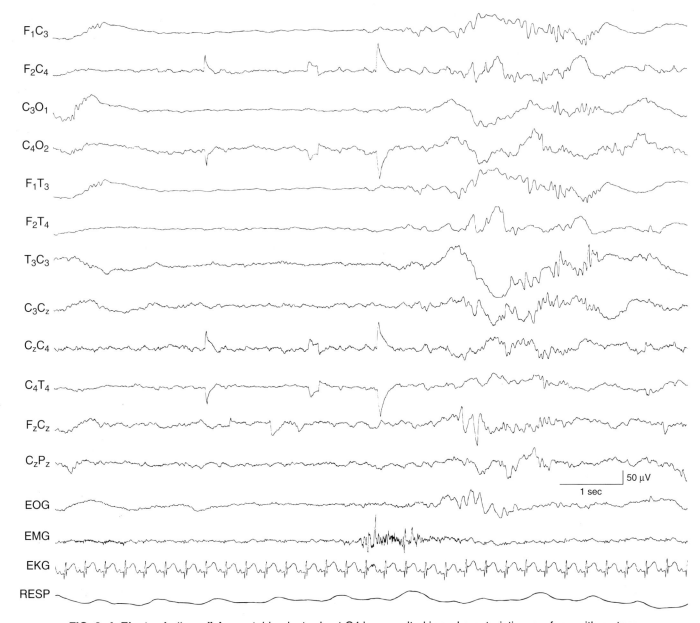

**FIG. 3–4. Electrode "pop."** An unstable electrode at C4 has resulted in a characteristic waveform with a steep initial component, sharp morphology, and more gradual return to baseline. This occurred in a 36-week CA infant whose background EEG is characterized by a suppression–burst pattern.

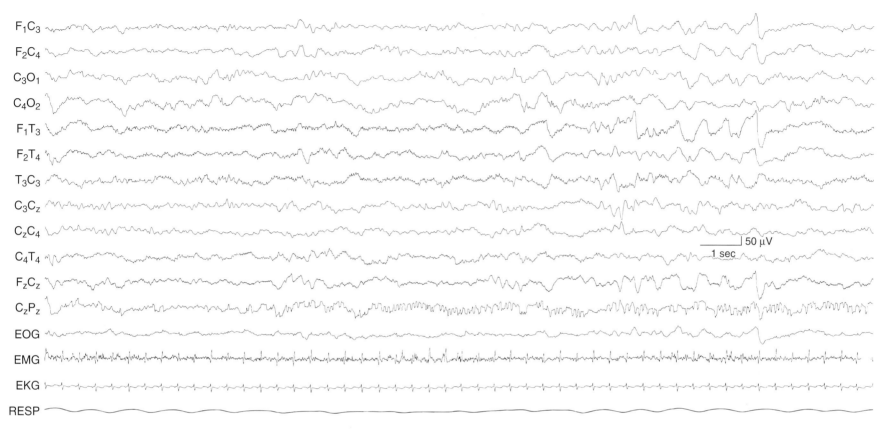

**FIG. 3–5. Irregular, sustained waveforms due to unstable electrode.** The Pz electrode in this recording has become unstable, resulting in irregular, sustained, low-voltage, relatively fast activity. Some of the waveforms have a nonphysiologic angular and square morphology. This occurred in a 42-week CA infant whose background EEG activity was normal.

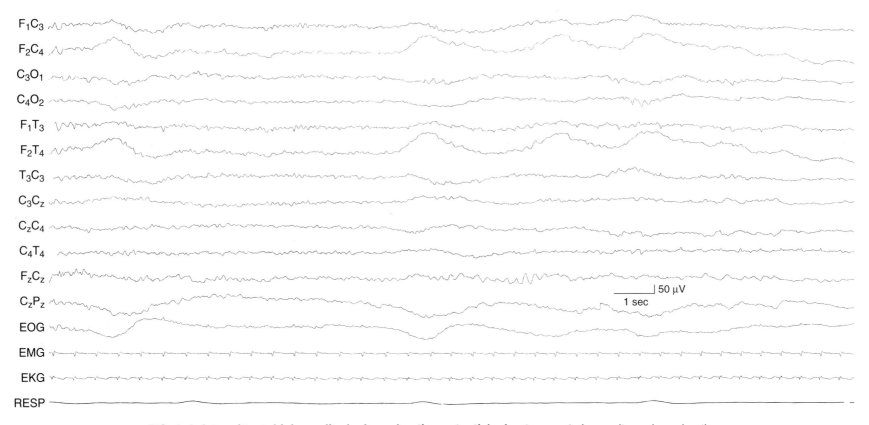

**FIG. 3–6. Intermittent, high-amplitude, long-duration potentials due to sweat.** Low-voltage, long-duration waveforms are present, predominantly in the right central region, because of excessive sweating in this 40-week CA infant with normal background EEG activity.

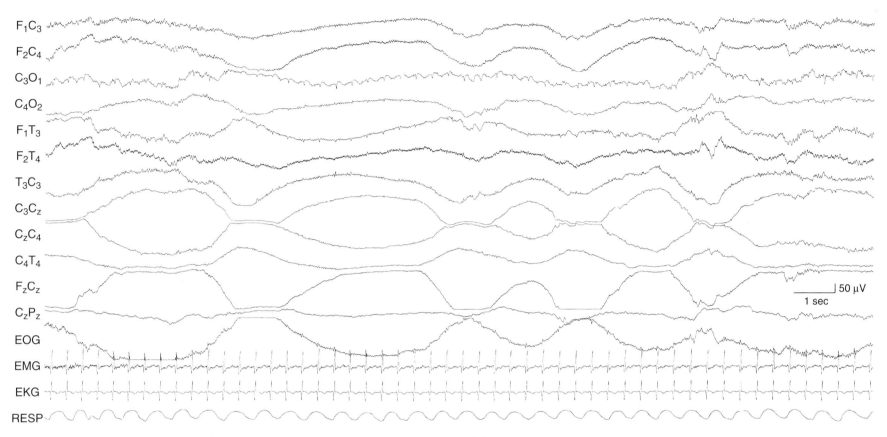

**FIG. 3–7. Sustained, high-amplitude, long-duration potentials due to sweat.** The high-voltage, long-duration waveforms are predominantly in frontal and central regions and are sustained. This activity is due to excessive sweating of the infant. The electrocardiogram also is reflected in leads from the left central region and there is electromyographic activity in the anterior leads. This infant is 40-week CA with a background EEG that is depressed and undifferentiated.

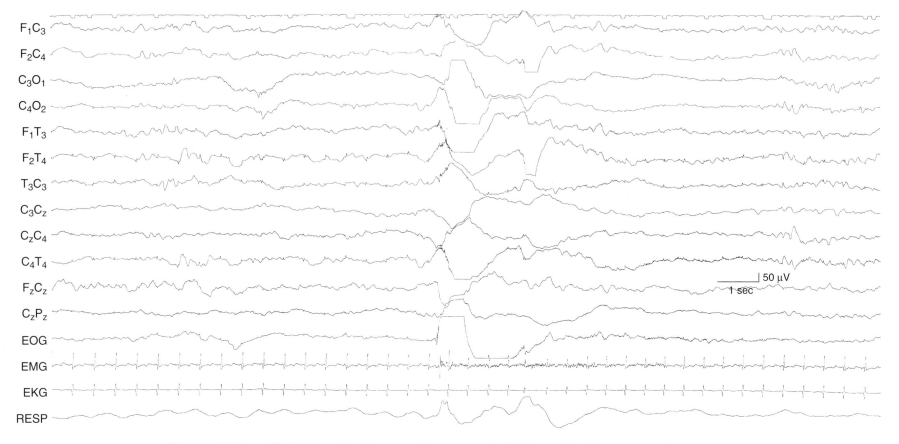

**FIG. 3–8. High-amplitude, long-duration, asynchronous potential due to head movement.** Spontaneous head movement has resulted in moderate-amplitude slow waves appearing in leads from both hemispheres, with some asynchronous components on the two sides in this 41-week CA infant with normal background EEG activity.

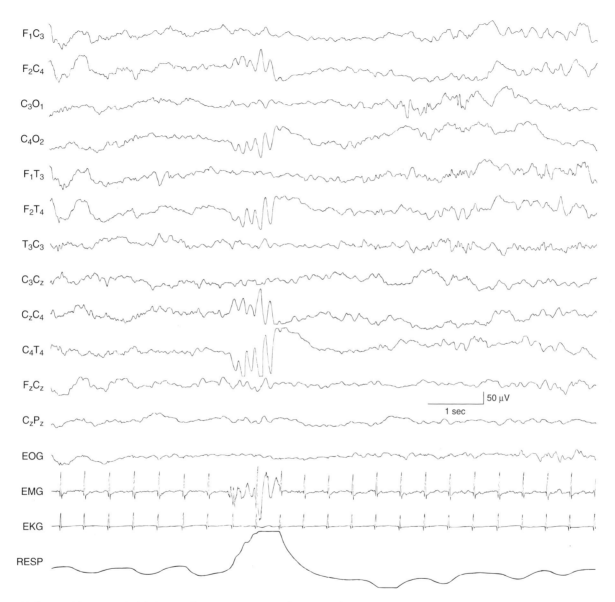

**FIG. 3–9. Moderately high-amplitude, short-duration, repetitive potentials due to head movement associated with sobbing.** This infant experienced a brief sobbing episode characterized by shuddering that involved respiration and truncal muscles as well as head, which was turned to the right. The rapid, rhythmic movement of the head resulted in brief rhythmic theta-like activity in the right central region in this 40-week CA infant with normal background EEG activity. The simultaneous body movements are indicated by waveforms in the electromyogram channel.

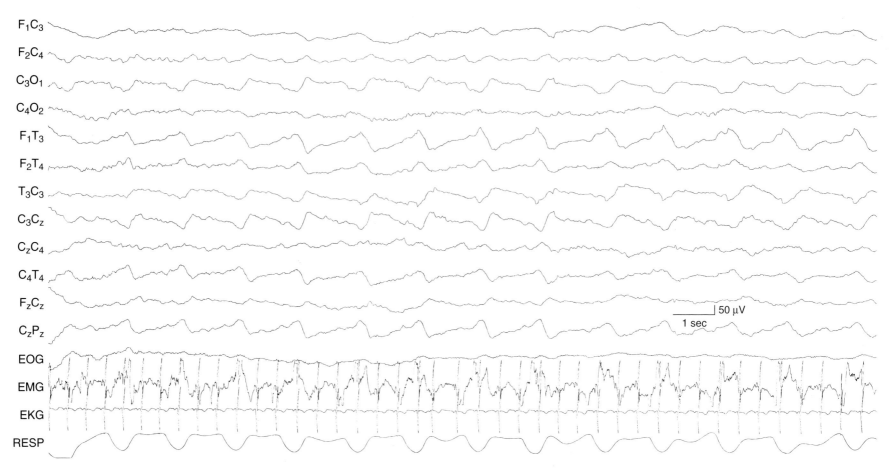

**FIG. 3–10. Slow periodic waves due to movements induced by mechanical ventilation.** Mechanical ventilation may produce movements of the body and head, which in turn may result in EEG artifact, as in this recording with periodic, very slow waveforms that are lateralized to left and are aligned with deflections in the respiration channel. The background EEG in this 40-week CA infant is depressed and undifferentiated.

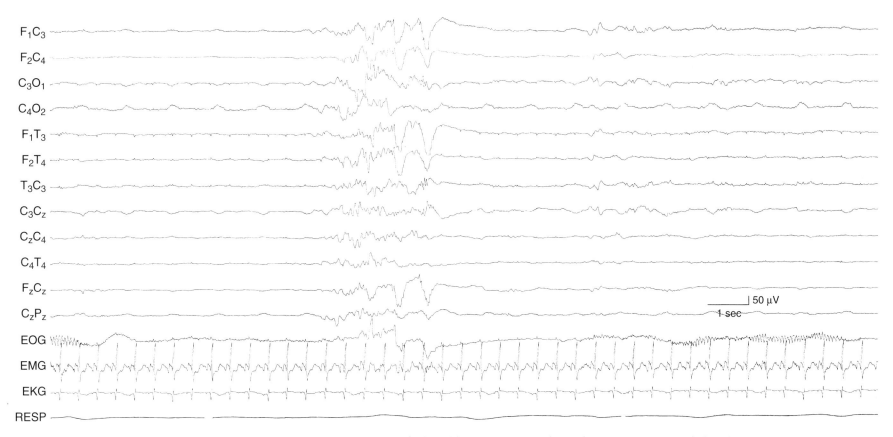

**FIG. 3–11. Periodic waves due to movement induced by extracorporeal membrane oxygenation (ECMO) pump.** Low-voltage, periodic waves primarily in the right occipital region are due to head movement induced by the action of the ECMO instrument used to support this 36-week CA infant. The background activity is characterized by a suppression-burst pattern.

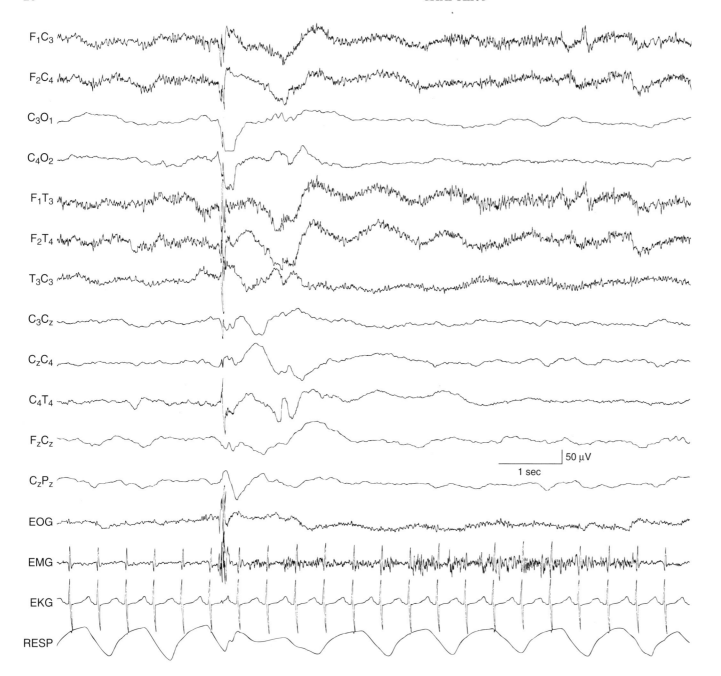

**FIG. 3–12. High-amplitude generalized spike-like artifact associated with generalized myoclonic movement.** A generalized myoclonic event in this 38-week CA infant resulted in a high-amplitude generalized spike-like waveform. Movement recorded as electromyographic (EMG) activity precedes the waveforms from scalp electrodes. There is sustained low-voltage EMG in the anterior leads.

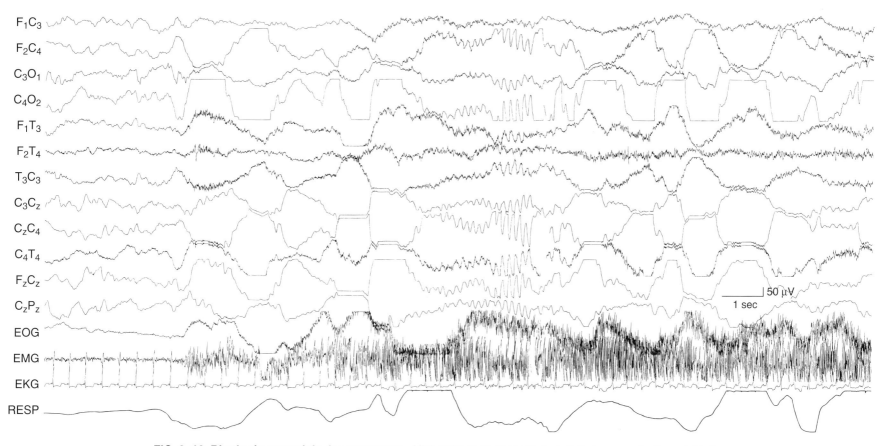

**FIG. 3–13. Rhythmic potentials due to tremors.** High-voltage rhythmic theta activity is present with variable lo-calization and is preceded and followed by high-voltage, very slow activity. This is due to this 44-week CA infant's tremulousness or jitteriness, preceded and followed by slow random movements of the body. Sustained elec-tromyographic activity is superimposed on the background EEG activity.

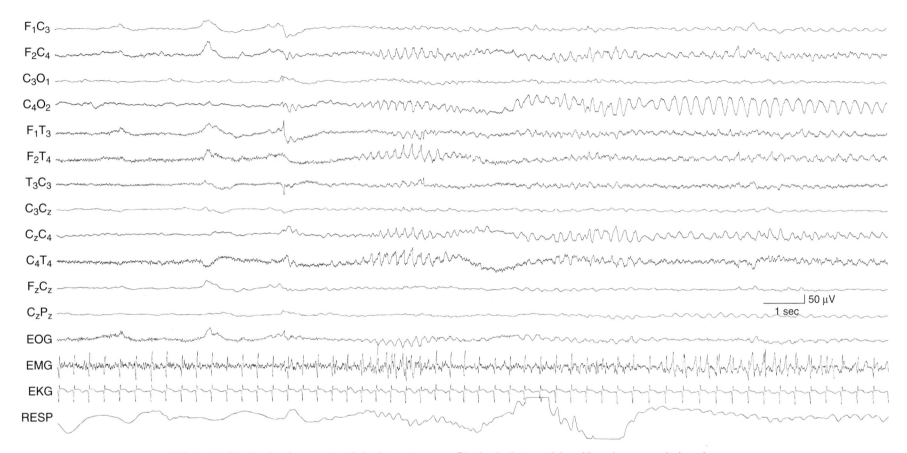

**FIG. 3–14. Rhythmic sharp potentials due to tremor.** Rhythmic theta activity with a sharp morphology is present in the right central region because of the tremors and jitteriness of the 40-week CA infant. Low-voltage electromyographic activity appears primarily in the temporal regions.

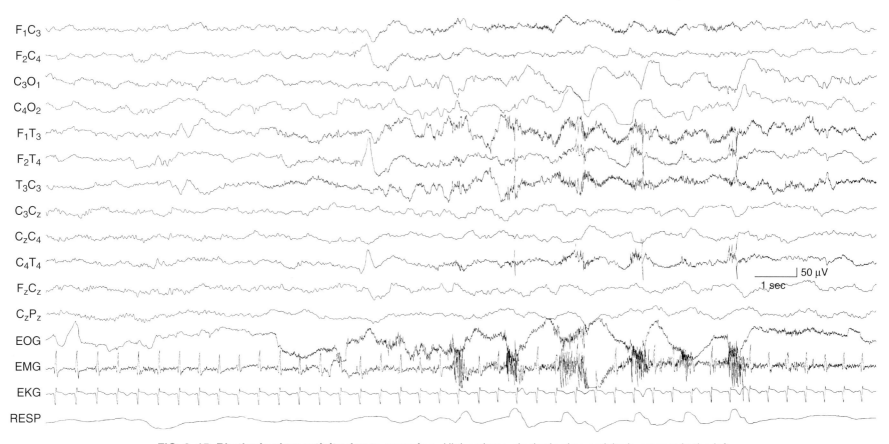

**FIG. 3–15. Rhythmic slow activity due to sneezing.** High-voltage, rhythmic slow activity is present in the left temporal region associated with repetitive sneezing or coughing of this 39-week CA infant with normal EEG background activity. Superimposed electromyographic (EMG) activity occurs in the EEG channels, and movement also is suggested by activity in the EMG channel.

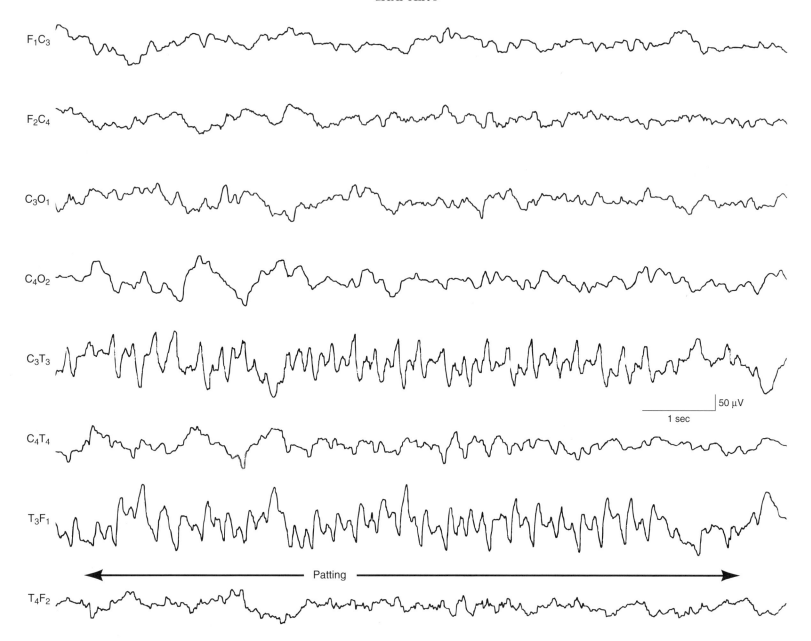

**FIG. 3–16. Rhythmic polymorphic activity induced by patting.** Polymorphic rhythmic activity in the left temporal region is induced by patting or comforting this 40-week CA infant with a normal background EEG.

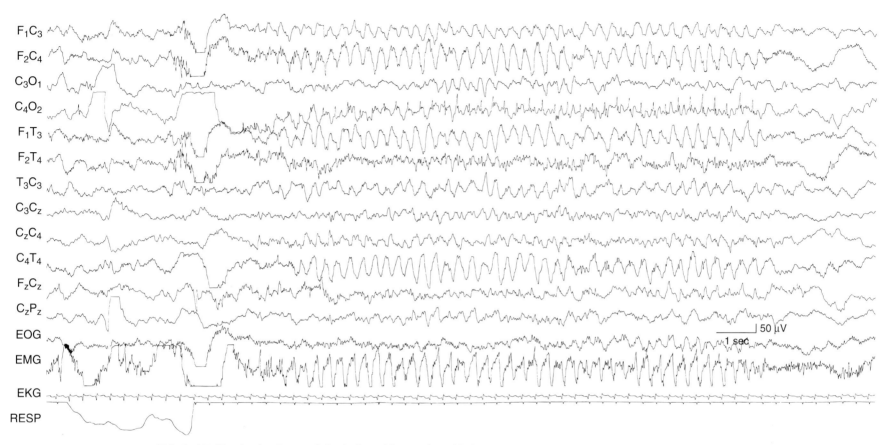

**FIG. 3–17. Rhythmic slow activity induced by patting.** High-voltage, rhythmic, monomorphic, delta-like activity is induced by patting this 40-week CA infant with normal EEG background activity.

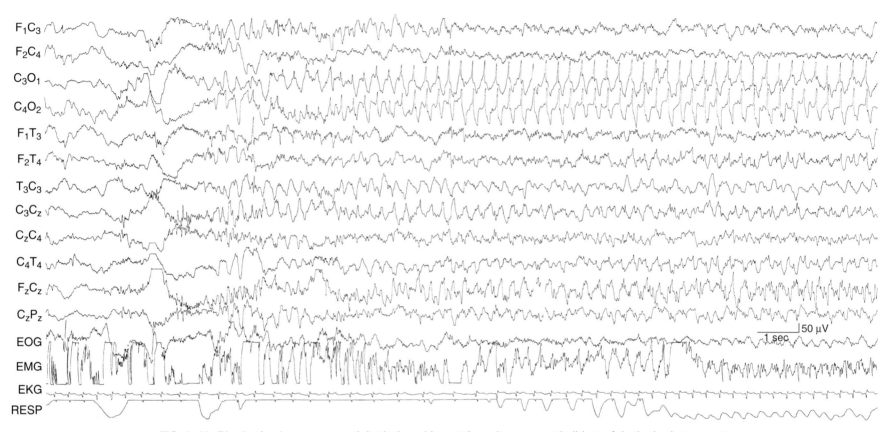

**FIG. 3–18. Rhythmic sharp wave activity induced by patting.** An apparent build-up of rhythmic sharp waves is present in the occipital regions bilaterally, with some lateralization to leads on the left, associated with patting of this 40-week CA infant. The background EEG activity is normal.

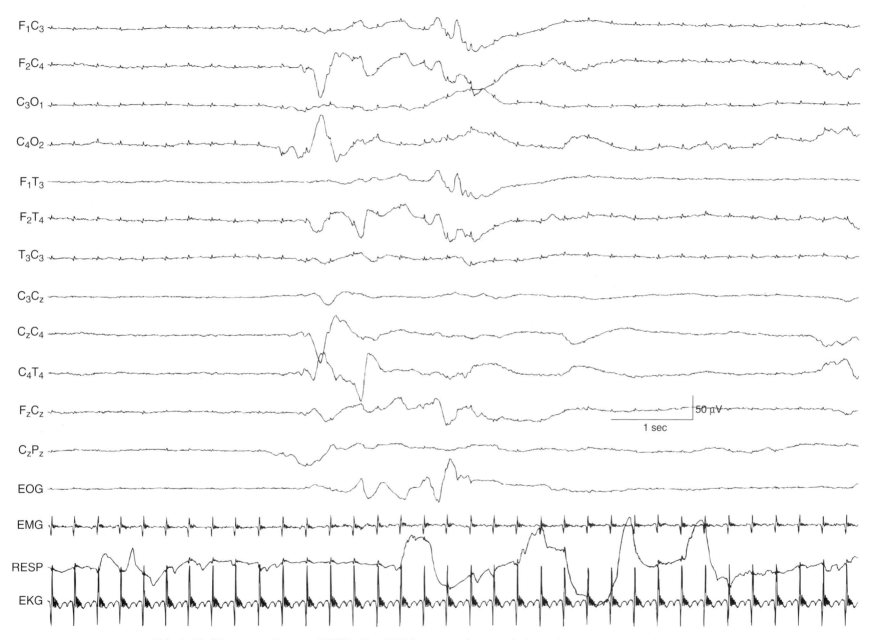

**FIG. 3–19. Electrocardiogram (EKG).** The EKG is present in several channels in this 39-week CA infant with suppression-burst EEG background activity.

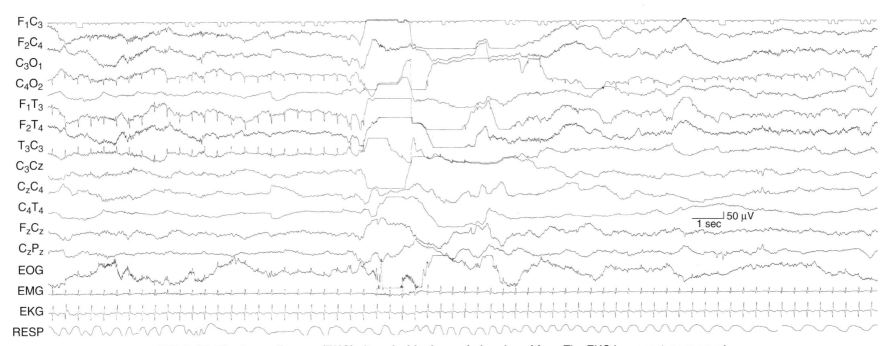

**FIG. 3–20. Electrocardiogram (EKG) altered with change in head position.** The EKG is present more prominently in the early portion of this recording, with high-amplitude spike-like activity in leads from the left occipital and temporal regions. The amplitude of the waves is reduced, and they are less prominent in the temporal region when the infant's head is moved to the midline by the technician. This movement is marked by the generalized high-amplitude slow activity in the middle of this segment. The infant is 40 weeks CA, and the background EEG activity is depressed and undifferentiated.

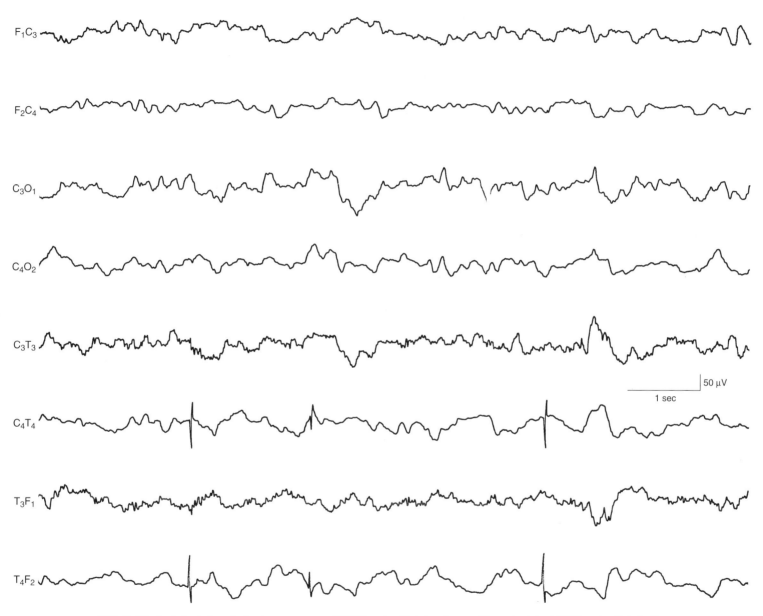

**FIG. 3–21. Isolated, focal electromyogram (EMG) potential due to sucking.** Isolated EMG potentials in the right temporal region result from sucking motions of this 40-week CA infant. The background EEG is within the range of normal variation.

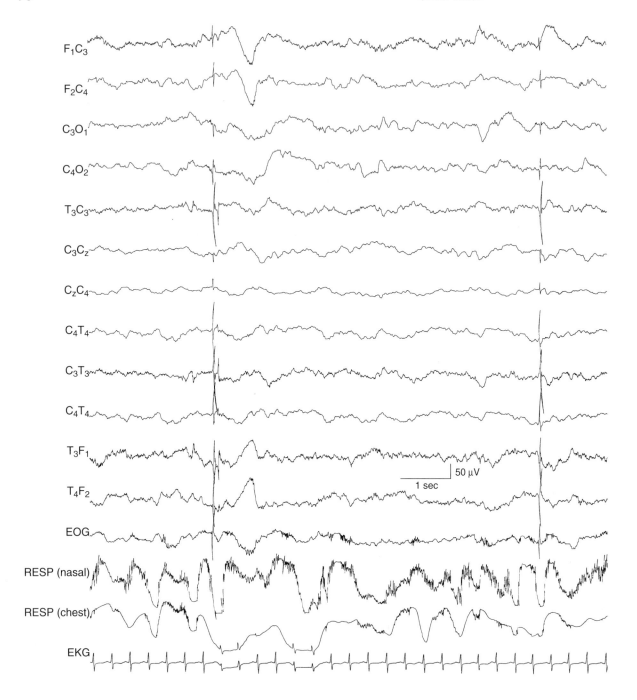

**FIG. 3–22. Wide reflection of electromyogram (EMG) potentials due to sucking.** The EMG due to sucking arises from the left temporal region but has variable amplitude and a wide reflection on the two sides in this 40-week CA infant with normal EEG background activity.

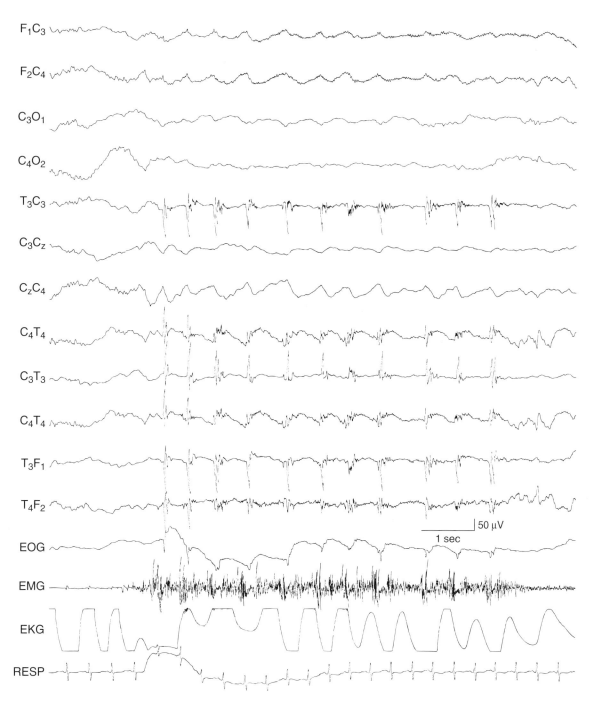

**FIG. 3–23. Periodic electromyogram (EMG) potentials due to sucking.** This EMG activity due to sucking has a complex morphology. It is periodic, primarily in the left temporal region. There is normal EEG background activity in this 40-week CA infant.

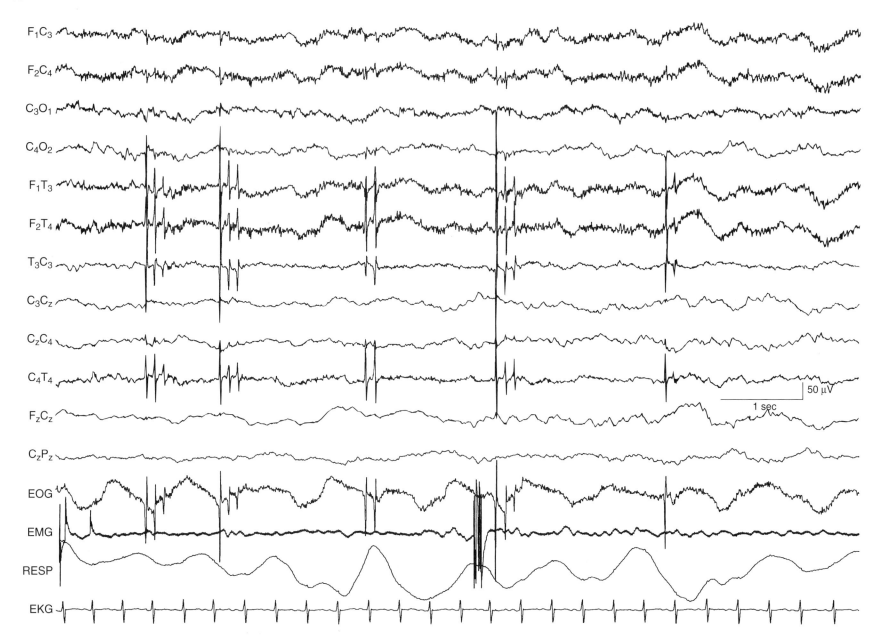

**FIG. 3–24. Periodic bursts of electromyogram (EMG) potentials due to sucking.** Brief bursts of repetitive EMG potentials occur periodically in the temporal regions bilaterally in this 41-week CA infant with normal EEG background activity. Low voltage, sustained EMG is present in anterior leads.

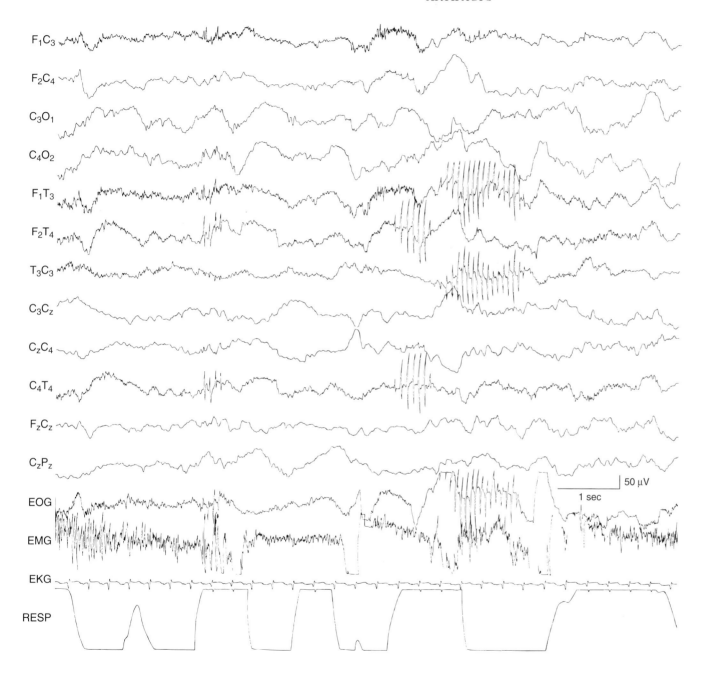

**FIG. 3–25. Multifocal, repetitive electromyogram (EMG) potentials due to jaw tremor.** Bursts of repetitive EMG due to tremulousness of the jaw are present independently in the left and right temporal regions in this 42-week CA infant with normal EEG background activity.

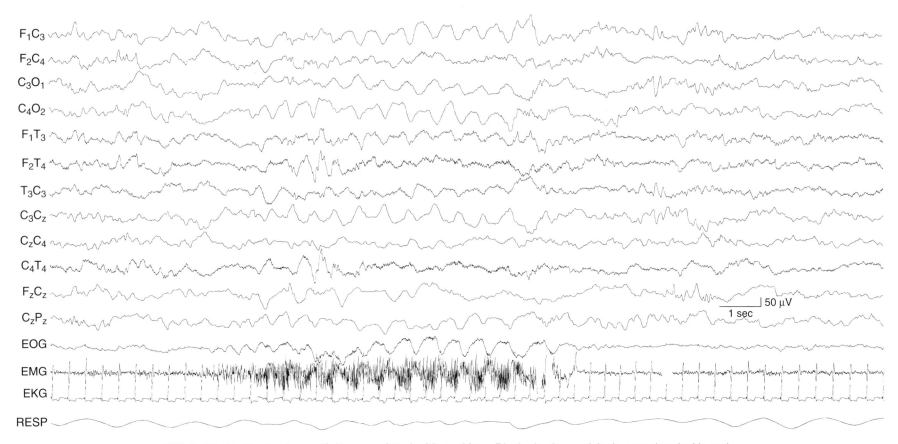

**FIG. 3–26. Rhythmic slow activity associated with sucking.** Rhythmic slow activity is associated with sucking in this 43-week CA infant. Although associated with sucking, this activity is not produced by endogenous potentials, but rather by movement of the head that occurs in conjunction with the vigorous sucking movements. The background EEG activity is within the range of normal variation. The electromyogram channel reflects increased activity associated with sucking.

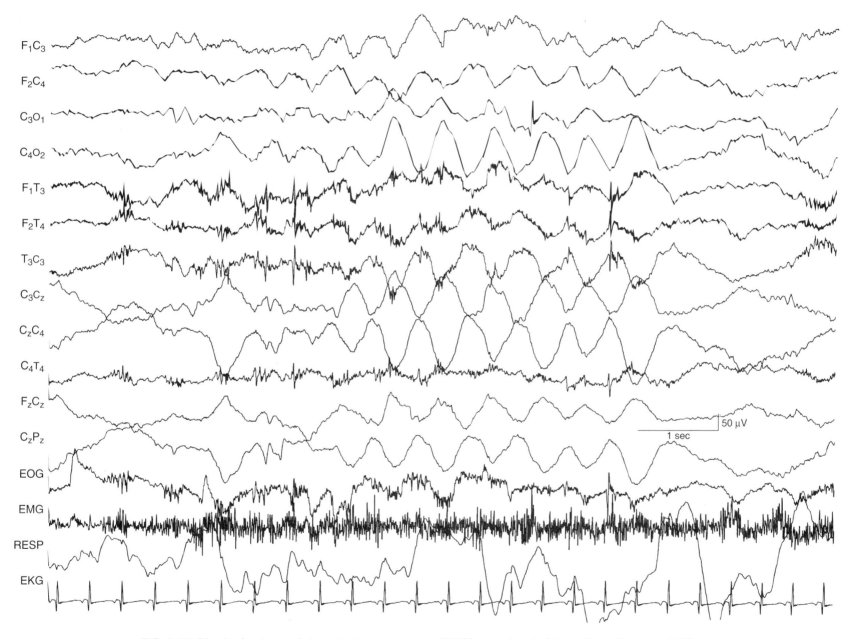

**FIG. 3–27. Rhythmic slow activity and electromyogram (EMG) associated with sucking.** Rhythmic EMG potentials are found in the temporal regions, and rhythmic slow activity is induced by head movement in the central regions associated with sucking in this 40-week CA infant with normal EEG background activity.

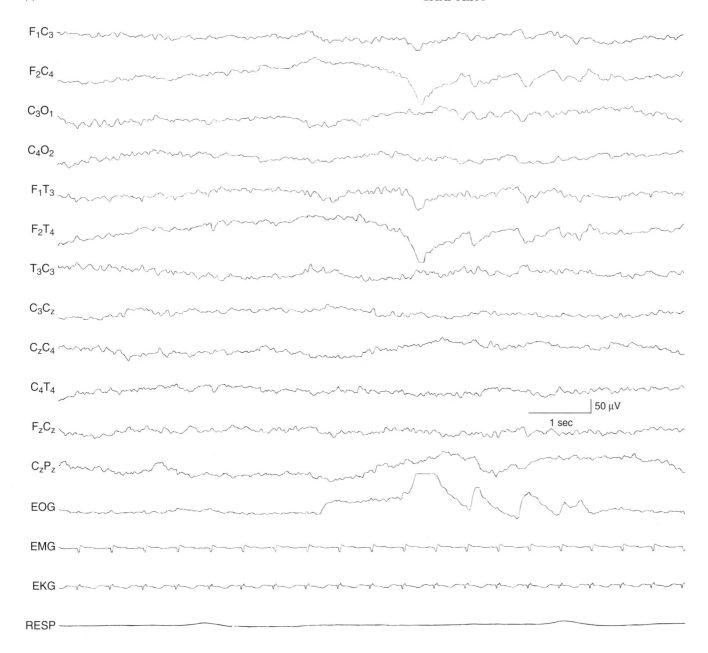

**FIG. 3–28. Slow activity due to eye movements.** A brief run of slow activity in the right frontal region aligns with the activity recorded in the electroculogram channel. The infant is 40 weeks CA with normal EEG background activity.

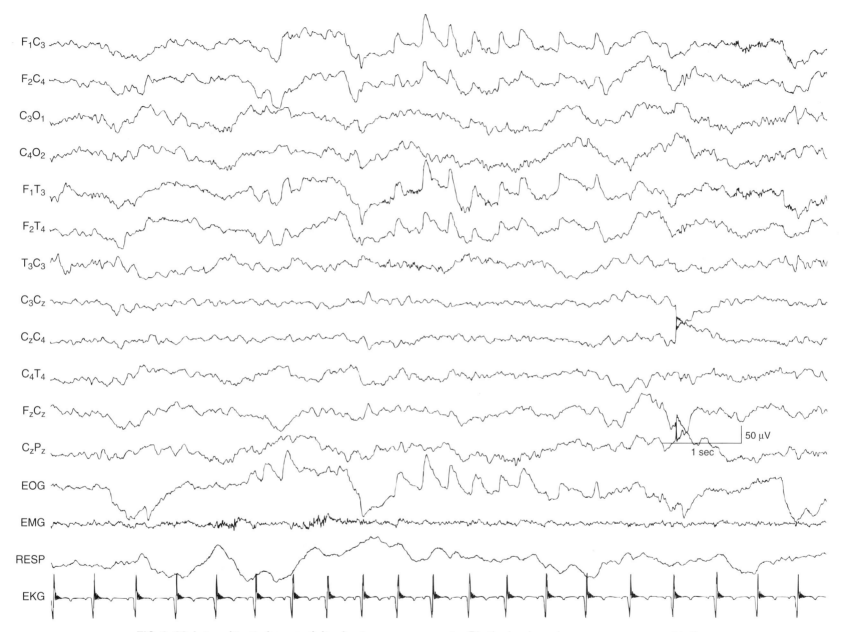

**FIG. 3–29. Intermittent sharp activity due to eye movements.** Rhythmic, slow, sharp waves are present in the frontal regions bilaterally, higher in amplitude on the left, aligned with the recorded electrooculogram and occurring in association with clinically observed nystagmus. The infant is 40 weeks CA with normal EEG background activity.

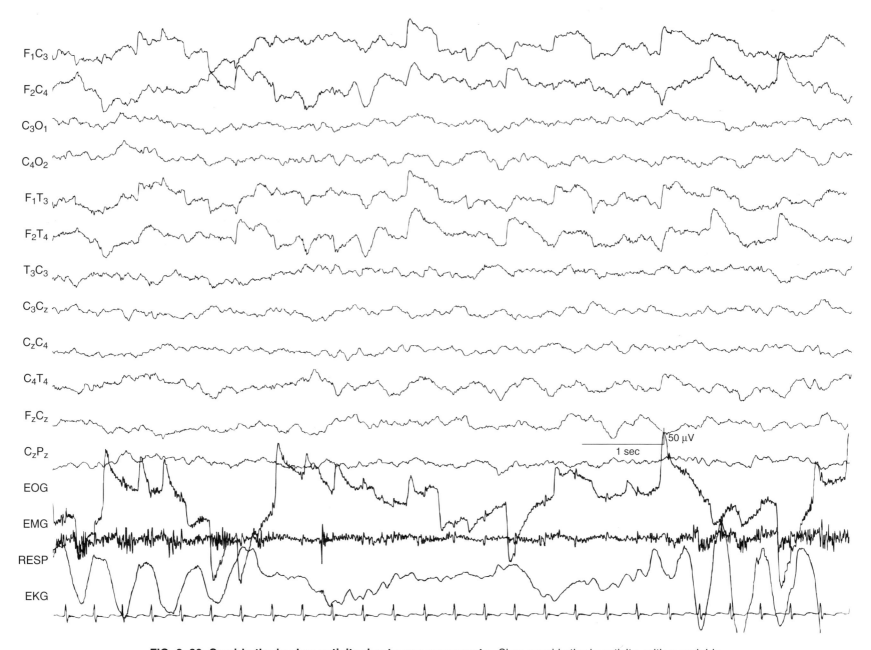

**FIG. 3–30. Semirhythmic slow activity due to eye movements.** Slow, semirhythmic activity, with a variable geometric morphology, is present in the frontal regions associated with eye movements that also are represented in the electrooculogram channel in the 40-week CA infant with normal EEG background activity.

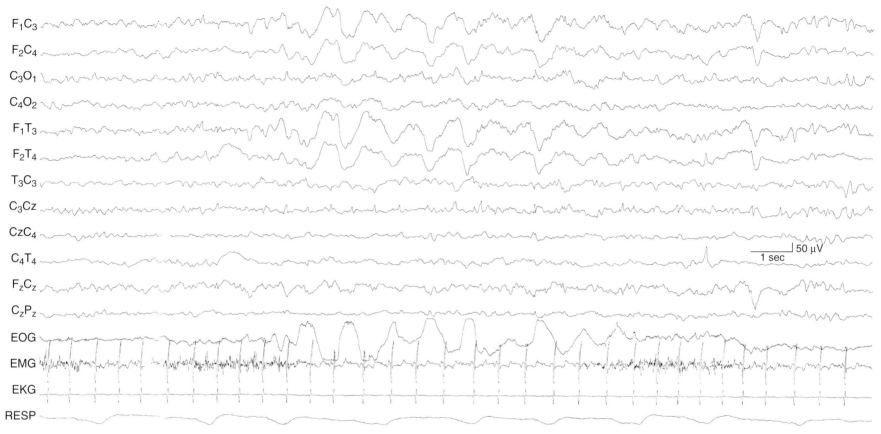

**FIG. 3–31. Slow activity associated with repetitive eye opening and closure.** High-voltage, slow activity is present in the frontal regions bilaterally associated with rhythmic eye opening and closure. This activity also is present in the electrooculogram channel. The EEG background activity is within the range of normal variation in this 39-week CA infant.

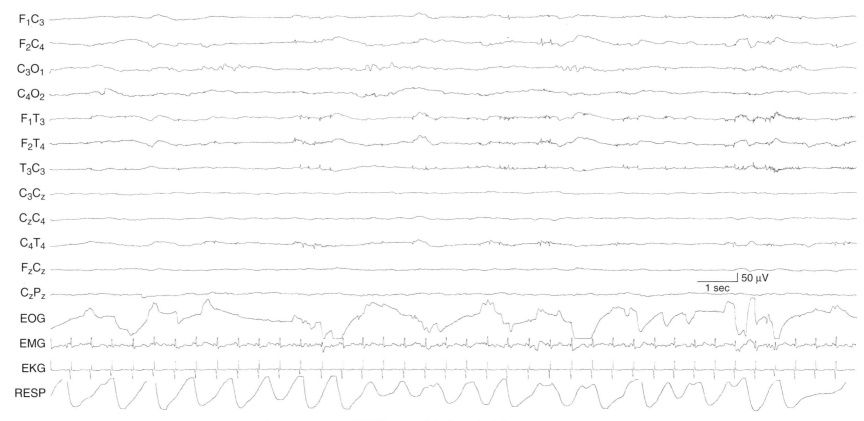

**FIG. 3–32. Random electromyogram (EMG) potentials from facial muscles.** Random low-voltage EMG potentials are present in the left and right temporal regions and, rarely, in the right frontal region, associated with twitches of facial muscles. The background activity is depressed and undifferentiated in this 41-week CA infant.

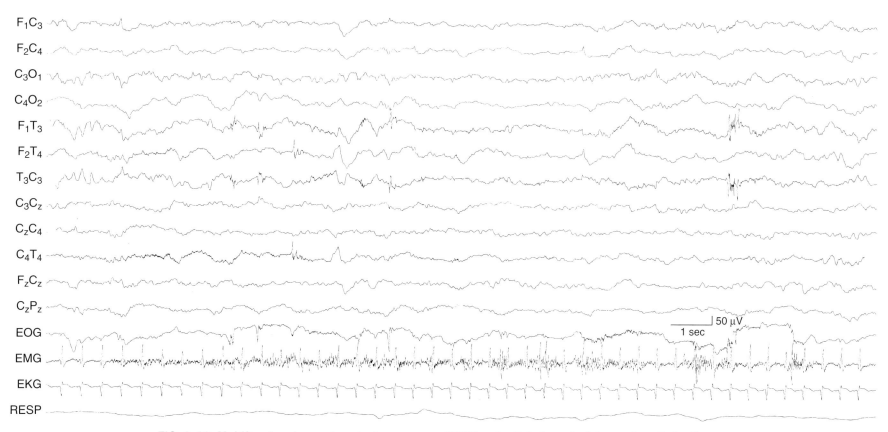

**FIG. 3–33. Multifocal and complex electromyogram (EMG) potentials from facial muscles.** Spike-like potentials are present in the left and right temporal regions, and a more complex burst of EMG activity is present later in the left temporal region in this 39-week CA infant with normal EEG background activity.

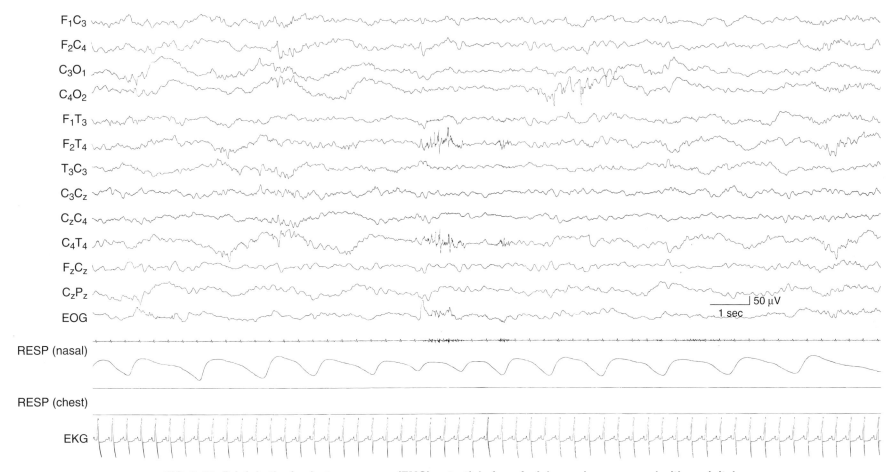

**FIG. 3–34. Brief rhythmic electromyogram (EMG) potentials from facial muscles compared with occipital sharp waves.** A burst of EMG activity is present in the right temporal region in the middle portion of this sample. In the latter portion of the recording, a burst of spike and sharp-wave activity of cerebral origin is present in the right occipital region (see Chapter 5) in this 39-week CA infant with otherwise normal EEG background activity.

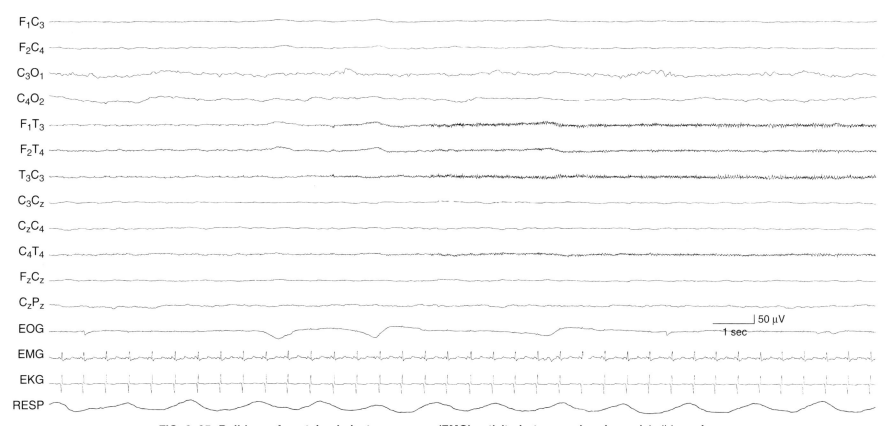

**FIG. 3–35. Build-up of sustained electromyogram (EMG) activity in temporal regions.** A build-up of sustained EMG activity is seen in the temporal regions bilaterally, higher in amplitude on the left. The background EEG is depressed and undifferentiated in the 41-week CA infant.

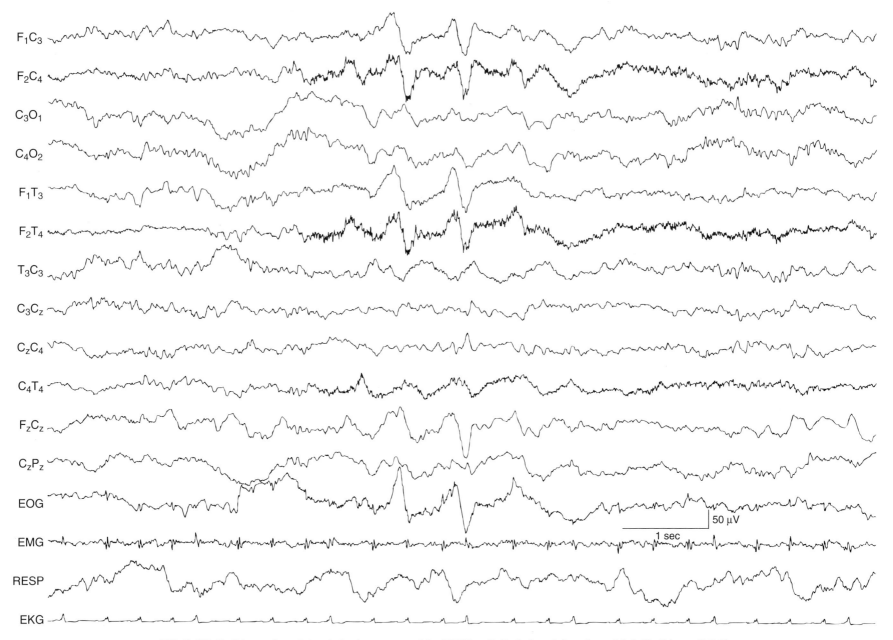

**FIG. 3–36. Build-up of sustained electromyographic (EMG) activity in frontal region.** A brief build-up of EMG activity is seen primarily in the right frontal region in this 37-week CA infant with normal EEG background activity.

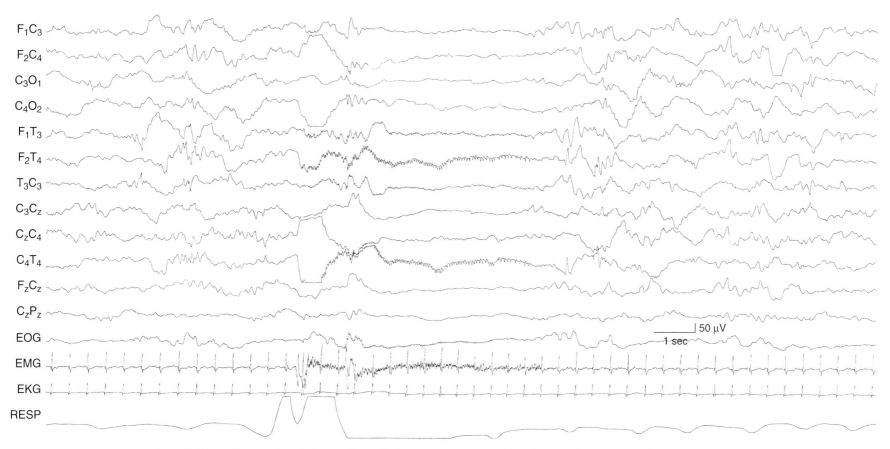

**FIG. 3–37. Build-up of sustained, slow electromyographic (EMG) activity in temporal region associated with arousal.** A burst of EMG activity is seen in the right temporal region with a relatively slow rate of firing. This activity occurs with the spontaneous arousal of the infant, associated on EEG with generalized voltage attenuation (see Chapter 4). The infant is 40 weeks CA with normal EEG background activity but with multifocal sharp waves of cerebral origin (see Chapter 5).

# CHAPTER 4

# Elements of the Normal Neonatal Electroencephalogram

Visual analysis of the neonatal electroencephalogram (EEG) requires the recognition of the conceptional age-dependent features characteristic of specific epochs of development. These electrographic features are presented here in four different formats: a table that lists specific elements (**Table 4–1**), a narrative that describes the continuum of development, and a summary by epoch of conceptional age (CA) of the expected elements. In addition, representative samples of EEG recordings in each epoch are provided.

Visual analysis and interpretation require determination of the degree of continuity of background activity (**Fig. 4–1**), and the degree of interhemispheric synchrony of the background activity (**Fig. 4–2**). They also require recognition of specific wave forms and patterns that occur with increasing age (**Fig. 4–3**), the appearance of sleep/wake cycles, and age-dependent response of the EEG to stimulation of the infant.

## CONTINUUM OF DEVELOPMENT

### Continuity

When the brain's electrical activity as revealed by the EEG first appears, it is discontinuous, with long periods of quiescence, and this pattern is referred to as *tracé discontinu* (Dreyfus-Brisac, 1956). As age increases, the periods of inactivity shorten (Anderson et al., 1985; Connell et al., 1978; Hahn et al., 1989; Selton et al., 2000). The longest acceptable single interburst-interval durations in relation to CA have been reported to be 26 weeks CA, 46 seconds; 27 weeks CA, 36 seconds; 28 weeks CA, 27 seconds (Selton et al., 2000); less than 30 weeks CA, 35 seconds; 31 to 33 weeks CA, 20 seconds; 34 to 36 weeks CA, 10 seconds; and 37 to 40 weeks CA, 6 seconds (Hahn et al., 1989; Clancy et al., 2003). At a CA of approx-

imately 30 weeks, continuous activity appears, but is present only during rapid eye movement (REM) sleep. At about 34 weeks CA, the EEG is predominantly continuous in the awake state. Continuity appears in non-REM (NREM) sleep at about 36 to 37 weeks CA. However, from that time until about 5 to 6 weeks after term, the EEG during periods of NREM sleep shows occasional episodes of generalized voltage, attenuation (not quiescence), lasting from 3 to 15 seconds; a pattern that has been called *tracé alternant* (Dreyfus-Brisac and Blanc, 1956). Examples of CA-dependent discontinuity are shown in **Figs. 4–4 to 4–31**.

### Bilateral Synchrony

Before 27 to 28 weeks CA, EEG activity occurs in generalized bisynchronous bursts (Selton et al., 2000). After 27 to 28 weeks CA, the activity is generally asynchronous in homologous regions of the hemispheres. The greater the distance from the midline, the greater the degree of asynchrony. With increasing maturity, the degree of asynchrony diminishes. The degree of asynchrony reflects not only maturation but also state. Thus asynchrony is most prominent in NREM sleep and is least prominent in REM sleep. The only exception to these general rules is that from the time frontal sharp waves first appear, at about 35 weeks CA, they are bilaterally synchronous. Examples of EEGs demonstrating CA-dependent synchrony are shown in **Figs. 4–4 to 4–31.**

### EEG Developmental Landmarks

An orderly appearance and disappearance of specific waveforms and patterns occurs with increasing CA (**Fig. 4–3**).

**TABLE 4–1.** *Developmental EEG characteristics of premature and term infants*

| Conceptional age (wk) | Continuity of background activity | | | Synchrony of background activity between homologous leads | | | EEG difference between wakefulness and sleep | Appearance and disappearance of specific waveforms and patterns | Reactivity to stimulus |
|---|---|---|---|---|---|---|---|---|---|
| | Awake | Quiet sleep | Active sleep | Awake | Quiet sleep | Active sleep | | | |
| 27–28 | — | D | D | — | ++++ | ++++ | No | | NR |
| 29–30 | D | D | D | 0 | 0 | 0 | No | 1. Temporal theta bursts (4–6 Hz)<br>2. Beta–delta complexes in central regions<br>3. Occipital very slow activity | NR |
| 31–33 | D | D | C | + | + | ++ | No | 1. Beta–delta complexes in occipitotemporal regions<br>2. Rhythmic 1.5-Hz activity in frontal leads in transitional sleep<br>3. Temporal alpha bursts replace 4- to 5-Hz bursts (33 wk) | NR |
| 34–35 | C | D | C | +++ | + | +++ | No | 1. Frontal sharp-wave transients<br>2. Extremely high voltage beta activity during beta–delta complexes<br>3. Temporal alpha bursts disappear | R |
| 36–37 | C | D | C | ++++ | ++ | ++++ | Yes | 1. Continuous bioccipital delta activity with superimposed 12- to 15-Hz activity during active sleep<br>2. Central beta–delta complexes disappear | R |
| 38–40 | C | C | C | ++++ | +++ | ++++ | Yes | 1. Occipital beta–delta complexes decrease and disappear by 39 wk<br>2. *Tracé alternant* pattern during NREM sleep | R |

D, discontinuous activity; C, continuous activity; ++++, total synchrony; 0, total asynchrony; NR, nonreactive; R, reactive; NREM, non–rapid eye movement.

From Hrachovy RA, Mizrahi EM, Kellaway P. Electroencephalography of the newborn. In: Daly DD, Pedley PA, eds. *Current practice of clinical neurophysiology*, 2nd ed. Philadelphia: Lippincott-Raven, 1991:202, with permission.

### *Beta–Delta Complexes*

These complexes constitute the prime landmarks of prematurity and are present from about 26 to 38 weeks CA. They consist of random 0.3- to 1.5-Hz waves of 50 to 250 μV, with superimposed bursts of low- to moderate-voltage fast activity. The frequency of the fast activity may vary, even in the same infant. Two frequencies predominate: 8 to 12 Hz and, more commonly, 18 to 22 Hz. The voltage of the fast activity varies throughout each burst but rarely exceeds 75 μV. **Figures 4–4 to 4–18** show typical beta–delta complexes at varying CAs. Various names have been given to these complexes: "spindle-delta bursts," "brushes," "spindle-like fast waves," and "ripples of prematurity." Dreyfus-Brisac and colleagues (1956), who first described the complexes, referred to them as "rapid bursts," emphasizing, as in other names, the fast component. An important feature of beta–delta complexes is that they typically occur asynchronously in derivations from homologous areas and show a variable voltage asymmetry on the two sides.

These complexes first appear as a dominant feature in the EEG at about 26 weeks CA. When first present they occur infrequently, largely in the central regions. During the next 5 to 6 weeks, they become progressively more persistent, and the voltage of the fast component usually increases. Until 32 weeks CA, the fast component has a predominant frequency of 18 to 22 Hz; thereafter, the slower frequency (8 to 12 Hz) is most often present. The spatial distribution of the

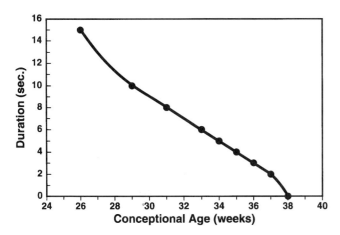

**FIG. 4–1. Average duration of discontinuous periods in NREM sleep in the EEG of the premature infant.** See text for details and references. (From Hrachovy RA. Development of the normal electroencephalogram. In: Levin KH, Luders HO, eds. *Comprehensive clinical neurophysiology.* Philadelphia: WB Saunders, 2000:387–413, with permission.)

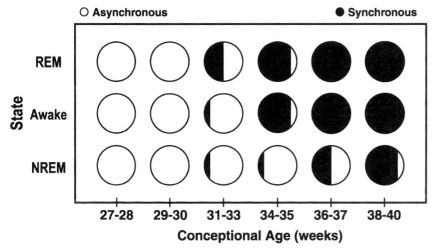

**FIG. 4–2. Development of interhemispheric synchrony in the EEG of the premature infant.** See text for details and references. Before 27–28 weeks CA, there are generalized bisynchronous bursts. (From Hrachovy RA. Development of the normal electroencephalogram. In: Levin KH, Luders HO, eds. *Comprehensive clinical neurophysiology.* Philadelphia: WB Saunders, 2000:387–413, with permission.)

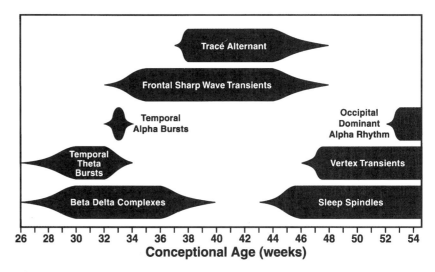

**FIG. 4–3. Appearance and disappearance of developmental EEG landmarks from prematurity to 3 months postterm.** See text for details and references. (From Hrachovy RA. Development of the normal electroencephalogram. In: Levin KH, Luders HO, eds. *Comprehensive clinical neurophysiology.* Philadelphia: WB Saunders, 2000:387–413, with permission.)

beta–delta complexes also changes with CA, becoming more prominent in the occipital and temporal areas with increasing age.

From the time beta–delta complexes first appear and changes in the wake/sleep cycle can be appreciated, the presence of beta–delta complexes is a prominent feature during REM sleep—a state characterized by virtually continuous EEG activity after 30 weeks CA. At 33 weeks CA, beta–delta complexes are maximally expressed in NREM sleep, rather than REM sleep, and appear more prominently in the temporooccipital areas. From 33 to 37 weeks CA, beta–delta complexes continue to occur primarily in NREM sleep.

### Temporal Theta and Alpha Bursts

A useful developmental marker is the appearance of rhythmic 4 to 6-Hz waves occurring in short bursts of rarely more than 2 seconds, arising independently in the left and right midtemporal areas. Voltage varies from roughly 20 to 200 μV. Individual waves may often have a sharp configuration (Hughes, 1987; Werner et al., 1977) (**Figs. 4–7, 4–8, 4–10, and 4–11**). This activity appears at about 26 weeks CA, is expressed maximally between 30 and 32 weeks, and then rapidly disappears. It is replaced by temporal alpha bursts that otherwise have characteristics of amplitude, burst duration, and spatial distribution as temporal theta bursts (**Figs. 4–12 to 4–14**). The presence of temporal alpha bursts is a very specific marker for 33 weeks CA, because they appear at the CA and are no longer present at 34 weeks CA.

### Frontal Sharp Waves

Frontal sharp waves are isolated sharp waves of blunt configuration, usually with an initial surface-negative phase followed by a surface-positive phase, and have been referred to as *encouche frontales* (Dreyfus-Brisac, 1962; Kellaway and Crawley, 1964). They may be present at 34 weeks CA but attain maximal expression at about 35 weeks CA. They diminish in number and voltage after 44 weeks CA and are only rarely seen in infants older than 6 weeks after term.

These frontal sharp transients are bilaterally synchronous and symmetrical from the time of their first appearance. The initial surface-negative component lasts about 200 milliseconds. The succeeding surface-positive component lasts somewhat longer, but this is quite variable and is often difficult to measure because intervening background activity obscures the termination of the waveform (**Figs. 4–15, 4–16, 4–20 to 4–23**). They typically occur randomly as single events, predominantly in transitional rather than in REM or NREM sleep. However, they also may recur in brief runs and may be mixed with another normal feature of near-term infants, bifrontal delta activity (**Fig. 4–23**).

### Distinguishing between the Waking and Sleep EEG

Until 36 to 37 weeks CA, distinguishing the various states of the wake/sleep cycle is based on empiric factors such as behavior and polygraphic parameters. Eye opening is associated with the awake state, and eye closure is associated with sleep. Regular respiration, random eye movements, and variable muscle tone are associated with NREM sleep, whereas irregular respiration, rapid eye movements, and decreased muscle tone are associated with REM sleep.

At about 30 weeks CA, the background activity is continuous in REM sleep and discontinuous during wakefulness and NREM sleep. However, the EEG activity in all states is characterized by the presence of beta–delta complexes and manifested according to their CA-dependent abundance, spatial distribution, and degree of synchrony (**Figs. 4–17 to 4–19**).

By 36 to 37 weeks CA, a clear distinction can be made between the waking EEG and the sleep EEG based on their inherent features, without reliance on clinical or polygraphic data (**Figs. 4–25 to 4–28**). In the awake EEG, beta–delta complexes are rarely present, and the awake background activity consists chiefly of continuous polyfrequency activity. This polyfrequency activity is characterized by random, very slow, low-voltage activity best described as baseline shifting, with superimposed semirhythmic 4- to 8-Hz activity in all regions. In addition, generalized, very low voltage 18- to 22-Hz activity and anteriorly distributed, very low voltage 2- to 3-Hz activity may be found. From the standpoint of determining CA, disappearance of the beta–delta complexes when the infant appears behaviorally awake constitutes an important marker of 38 weeks CA.

Before about 36 weeks CA, the background activity in NREM sleep is discontinuous (**Fig. 4–18**). Between 36 and 38 weeks CA, two NREM EEG patterns emerge. The first is continuous high-voltage, slow-wave activity in all regions. The second pattern is known as *tracé alternant* and is characterized by a modulation of activity with alternating periods of high- and low-voltage activity (**Fig. 4–27**). This pattern may occur in infants through 44 weeks CA. After that period, NREM sleep is characterized by continuous slow-wave activity with the eventual emergence of sleep spindles after about 46 weeks CA, although rudimentary spindles may occur earlier (**Figs. 4–30 and 4–31**).

The terms *transitional sleep* and *indeterminant sleep* are used to characterize the state of the infant when it cannot be precisely determined by specific EEG criteria.

### Reactivity to Stimulation

Changes in EEG activity in response to stimuli do not clearly emerge until about 33 to 34 weeks CA (**Fig. 4–19**), and by 37 weeks of CA, these responses can be easily elicited.

The response to a stimulus is related to the character of the ongoing activity at the time of the stimulus. If high-voltage, very slow activity is present, an effective stimulus produces abrupt and pronounced generalized attenuation of voltage lasting as long as 5 to 10 seconds. A pattern less often seen may occur if the background activity is of low voltage, with predominant theta activity; then an effective stimulus may elicit high-voltage, generalized delta waves lasting 5 to 15 seconds (Ellingson, 1958; Kellaway and Crawley, 1964).

Spontaneous episodes of attenuation may be associated with self-arousal (**Fig. 4–29**). They occur in infants until about 2 weeks after term, possibly in response to interoceptive stimuli. Such episodes should not be interpreted as evidence of immaturity or be confused with the repetitive episodes of generalized or regional attenuation that may occur in abnormal conditions of diffuse cerebral dysfunction, such as neonatal hypoxic–ischemic encephalopathy.

## Special Waveforms and Patterns

Some special waveforms and patterns, particularly in the near-term and term infant, are considered to be within the range of normal variation, although they are not developmental milestones *per se*. They are bifrontal delta activity and some forms of temporal sharp waves.

### *Bifrontal Delta Activity*

Bifrontal delta activity appears in the near-term or term infant as intermittent rhythmic 1.5- to 2-Hz high-voltage activity in the frontal regions bilaterally (**Fig. 4–23**). This activity may occur in close association with frontal sharp transients, most prominently during transitional sleep. This pattern, characterized by bifrontal delta activity, has been referred to as "anterior dysrhythmia." However, this is a misnomer, because it does not suggest abnormality and is considered within the range of normal variation (Clancy et al., 2003).

### *Temporal Sharp Waves*

Temporal sharp waves are discussed in detail in the following chapter that concerns findings of uncertain diagnostic significance. That discussion describes criteria used to differentiate normal temporal sharp waves from those that are clearly abnormal. Temporal sharp waves that have a simple diphasic morphology, with the initial component appearing as surface-negative in polarity, that occur randomly and that usually appear asynchronously on the two sides and during sleep can be considered normal (**Fig. 4–24**). Complex morphology, positive polarity, persistent localization, and occurrence during wakefulness are criteria for abnormality.

## SUMMARY OF CONCEPTIONAL AGE–DEPENDENT FINDINGS

### 24 to 26 Weeks Conceptional Age

**Continuity.** There are brief bursts of activity between periods of electrical quiescence. The interburst interval is CA dependent and has its longest duration at this age.
**Synchrony.** Bursts of activity during this epoch are synchronous on the two sides.
**Landmarks.** Beta–delta complexes are present during this epoch.

**Wake/sleep cycles.** Cycles are not well defined by behavior or polygraphic changes. No evidence is seen of wake/sleep cycling on EEG.
**Reactivity.** No reactivity to stimulation occurs.

### 27 to 28 Weeks Conceptional Age (Figs. 4–4 and 4–5)

**Continuity.** Electrical activity is episodic. Brief periods of generalized moderate-voltage activity may appear between periods of generalized electrical quiescence. The interburst interval is relatively long compared with that present at later ages.
**Synchrony.** The bursts of electrical activity are asynchronous on the two sides.
**Landmarks.** Beta–delta complexes are present in the central regions, and rudimentary temporal theta bursts are present.
**Wake/sleep cycles.** Cycles are not well defined by behavior or polygraphic changes. No evidence of wake/sleep cycles is found on EEG.
**Reactivity.** No reaction to stimulation occurs.

### 29 to 30 Weeks Conceptional Age (Figs. 4–6 to 4–9)

**Continuity.** The EEG remains discontinuous. Although brief periods occur in which behavioral and physiologic parameters suggest REM sleep, the EEG activity is relatively continuous. The duration of the interburst intervals is less than that in preceding epochs.
**Synchrony.** Asynchrony between the two hemispheres is a predominant feature.
**Landmarks.** Beta–delta complexes are present in the central regions. Temporal theta bursts are a consistent feature during this epoch. Occipital slow (delta) activity emerges during this epoch.
**Wake/sleep cycles.** The EEG is continuous during periods when behavioral and physiologic parameters indicate REM sleep. No clear-cut relation is seen between the stages of wakefulness and sleep on EEG activity except for a tendency for greater continuity of the background activity during REM sleep.
**Reactivity.** No reaction to stimulation occurs.

### 31 to 33 Weeks Conceptional Age (Figs. 4–10 to 4–14)

**Continuity.** Continuous activity remains an aspect of REM sleep, but the EEG is discontinuous at other times.
**Synchrony.** The degree of synchrony between hemispheres increases; however,

this epoch is still marked by asynchrony when compared with epochs of infants at later ages.

**Landmarks.** Beta–delta complexes are present and are more prominent in the occipital and temporal regions than in the central regions. Temporal *theta* bursts persist until 32 weeks CA and are largely replaced by temporal *alpha* bursts at 33 weeks CA, which, in turn, disappear by 34 weeks CA.

**Wake/sleep cycles.** The EEG is continuous during REM sleep and discontinuous during wakefulness and NREM sleep.

**Reactivity.** No reaction to stimulation occurs.

### 34 to 35 Weeks Conceptional Age (Figs. 4–15 to 4–18)

**Continuity.** During wakefulness and REM sleep, the EEG is continuous, but is still discontinuous during NREM sleep, although the degree of discontinuity is less than that during the previous epoch.

**Synchrony.** Synchrony continues to be greater during this epoch than in early epochs, but asynchrony persists, chiefly in NREM sleep.

**Landmarks.** Frontal sharp transients (*encouche frontales*) become well defined by week 35 CA, although they may appear in rudimentary form during the week 34 CA. During this epoch, beta–delta complexes persist. Temporal alpha bursts disappear by 34 weeks CA.

**Wake/sleep cycles.** The EEG is continuous during wakefulness and REM sleep, but discontinuous during NREM sleep.

**Reactivity.** The background activity is reactive to stimulation of the infant. The response and its character are dependent on the state of the infant at the time of stimulation (**Figs. 4–10 and 4–29**).

### 36 to 37 Weeks Conceptional Age (Figs. 4–19 and 4–20)

**Continuity.** During wakefulness and REM sleep, the EEG is continuous, but episodes of discontinuity may occur in NREM sleep.

**Synchrony.** Synchrony continues to be greater during this epoch than in early epochs, now with most of activity synchronous on the two sides.

**Landmarks.** Frontal sharp transients persist. During this epoch, beta–delta complexes become less frequent. No new characteristic waveforms emerge, although bifrontal delta activity (a normal phenomenon) may be present during this epoch.

**Wake/sleep cycles.** EEG and physiologic features of wakefulness, REM sleep, and NREM sleep are seen. At 36 weeks CA, a clear distinction can be made, based on EEG criteria, between wakefulness and NREM sleep.

**Reactivity.** The background is reactive to stimulation.

### 38 to 40 Weeks Conceptional Age (Figs. 4–21 to 4–29)

**Continuity.** The EEG is continuous in all states of sleep and in wakefulness.

**Synchrony.** All activity becomes synchronous on the two sides by 40 weeks CA.

**Landmarks.** Frontal sharp transients persist. During this epoch, beta–delta complexes disappear from NREM sleep and are not present after 38 weeks CA.

**Wake/sleep cycles.** EEG and physiologic features of wakefulness, REM sleep, and NREM sleep are present. During this epoch, during NREM sleep, a modulation of the amplitude of the slow activity occurs with alternating periods of high and low voltage (*tracé alternant*) (**Fig. 4–27**).

**Reactivity.** The background is reactive to stimulation.

### 41 to 44 Weeks Conceptional Age (Fig. 4–30)

**Continuity.** The EEG is continuous in wakefulness and all stages of sleep.

**Synchrony.** Synchrony is virtually complete, as in the previous epoch.

**Landmarks.** Frontal sharp transients persist. No other immature waveforms are present.

**Wake/sleep cycles.** All stages of sleep and wakefulness are present. *Tracé alternant* begins to resolve by 44 weeks CA. NREM sleep is otherwise characterized by continuous slow-wave activity. Toward the end of this epoch, rudimentary sleep spindles may appear (**Fig. 4–30**). By 46 weeks CA, they are seen in all infants (**Fig. 4–31**).

**Reactivity.** The background is reactive to stimulation.

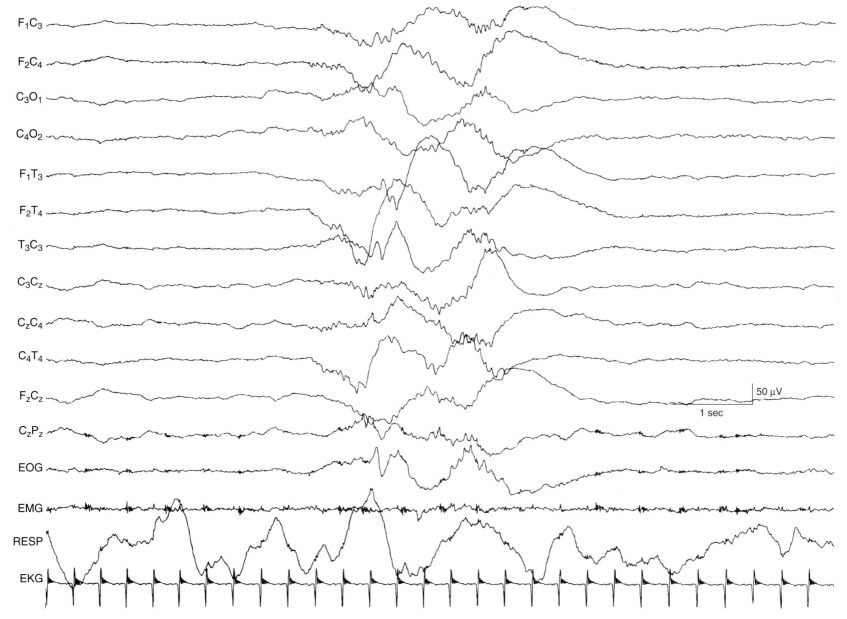

**FIG. 4–4. 26 to 27 weeks CA. *Tracé discontinu* and a burst of bilaterally synchronous, polyfrequency activity.** The EEG demonstrates a *tracé discontinu* pattern. A burst of bilaterally symmetrical, somewhat asynchronous activity is present. This activity is slow, with superimposed waves of faster frequency that resemble beta–delta complexes.

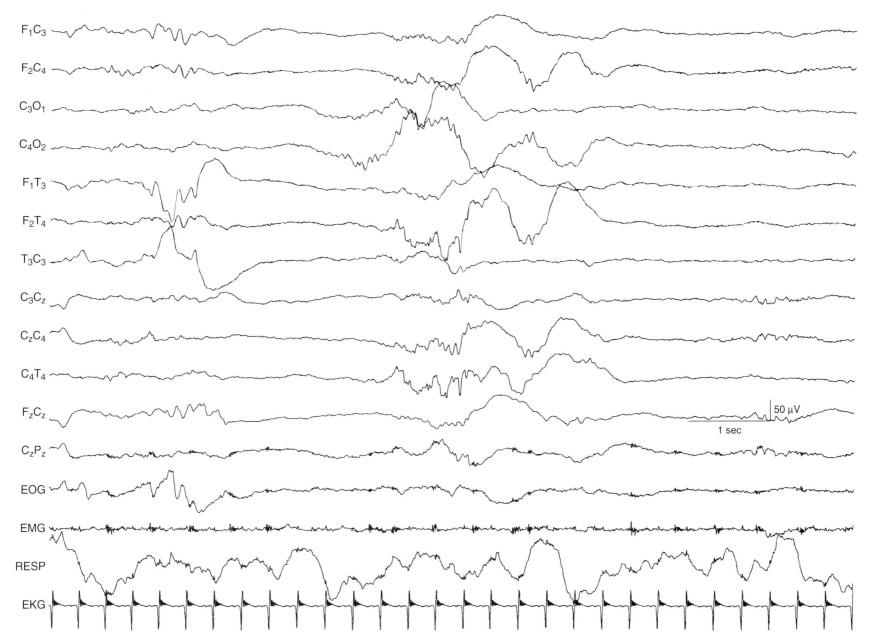

**FIG. 4–5. 27 to 28 weeks CA. Central beta–delta complexes.** The background is characterized by *tracé discontinu.* Beta–delta complexes are present, predominantly in the right central region.

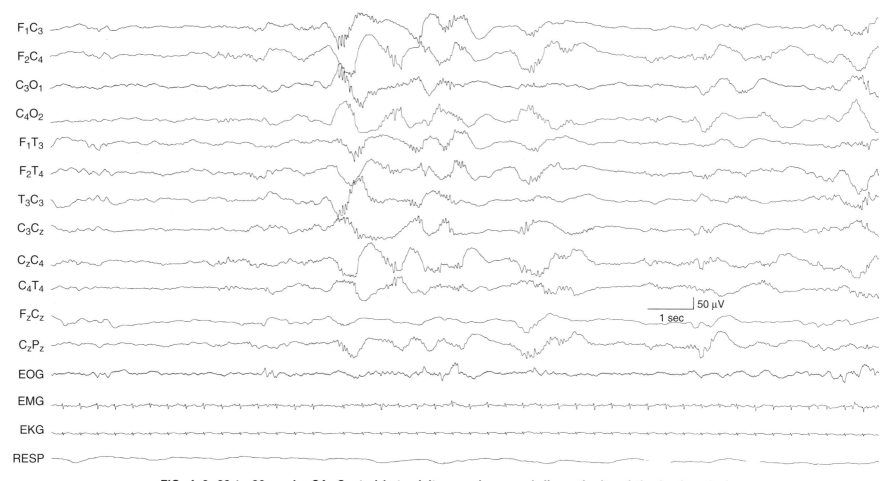

**FIG. 4–6. 29 to 30 weeks CA. Central beta–delta complexes and discontinuity of the background.**
Beta–delta complexes are present in the central regions bilaterally, but occur asynchronously on the two sides. The background activity is discontinuous with some low-voltage activity superimposed.

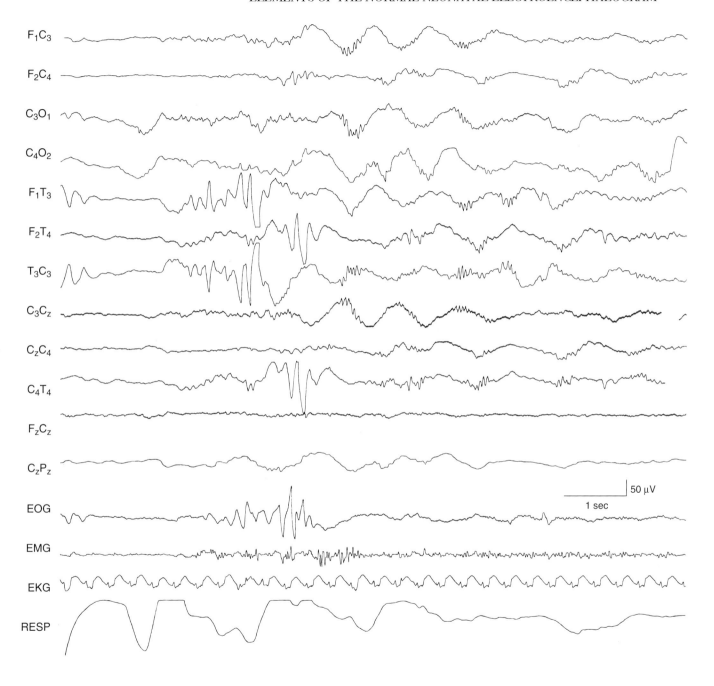

**FIG. 4–7. 29 to 30 weeks CA. Central beta–delta complexes and temporal theta bursts.** Theta bursts are present independently on the right and left temporal regions. Beta–delta complexes are present bilaterally, although asynchronous and more prominent on the left.

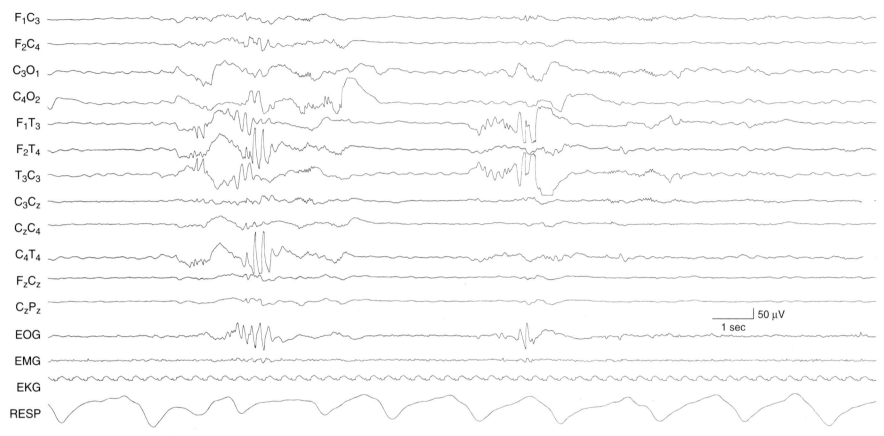

**FIG. 4–8. 29 to 30 weeks CA. Bilateral, independent temporal theta bursts.** Temporal theta bursts are present bilaterally, but independently. The background activity is discontinuous. The low-voltage rhythmic slow activity present during periods of quiescence is electrocardiogram artifact. This sample is from the same recording as in Fig. 4–9.

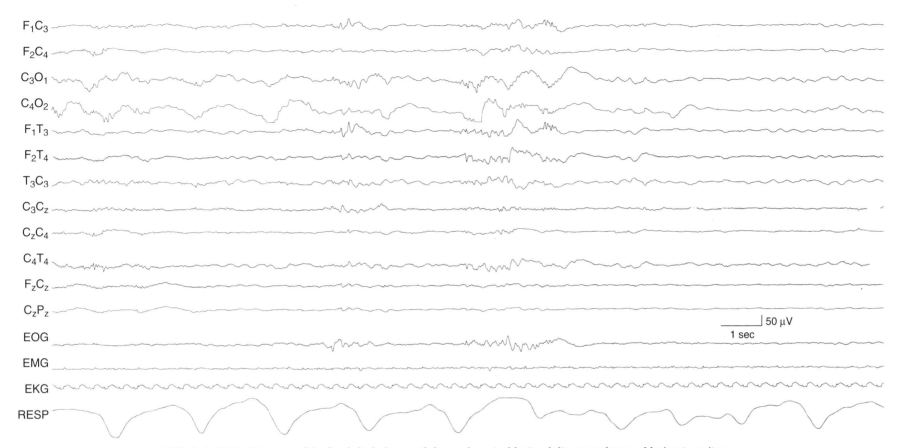

**FIG. 4–9. 29 to 30 weeks CA. Occipital slow activity and central beta–delta complexes.** Moderate-voltage, very slow activity appears in the occipital regions bilaterally in the early portion of the sample. Beta–delta complexes that are more central in location are present later. The recording then becomes discontinuous, with ECG artifact superimposed. This sample is from the same recording as that in Fig. 4–8.

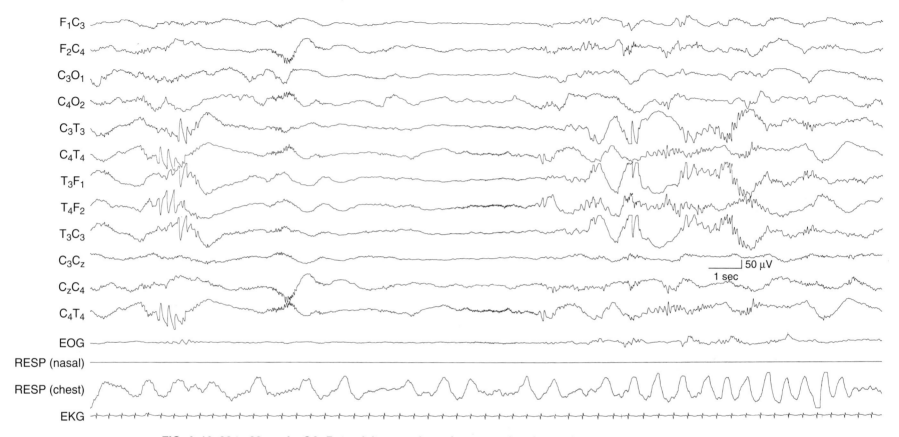

**FIG. 4–10. 30 to 32 weeks CA. Beta–delta complexes in temporal region and temporal theta bursts.** Beta-delta complexes are present in the temporal regions in the latter half of the sample. Earlier a beta–delta complex is seen in the right central region, with theta bursts in the temporal regions bilaterally, but asynchronously. The background activity is discontinuous.

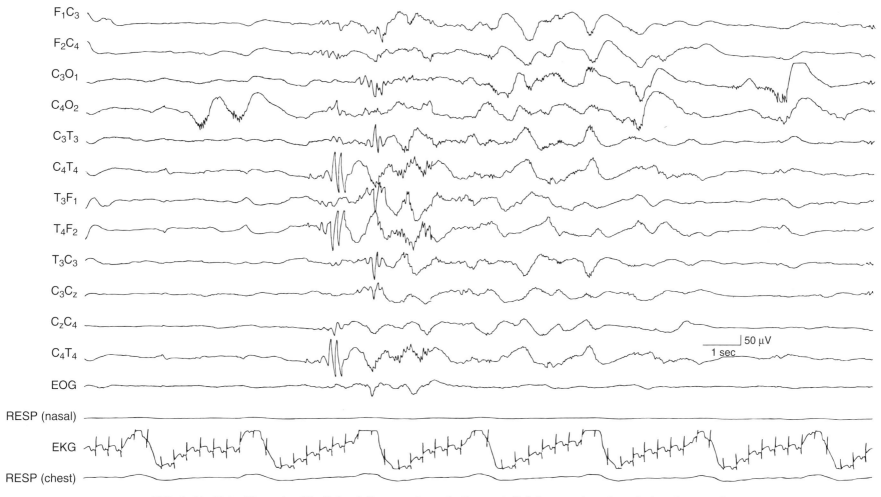

**FIG. 4–11. 30 to 32 weeks CA. Beta–delta complexes in the occipital, temporal, and central regions and temporal theta bursts.** In the early portion of the sample, a beta–delta complex is present in the right occipital region, and then bilateral, independent temporal theta bursts appear. Later, beta–delta complexes are found in the central regions bilaterally. The background activity is discontinuous.

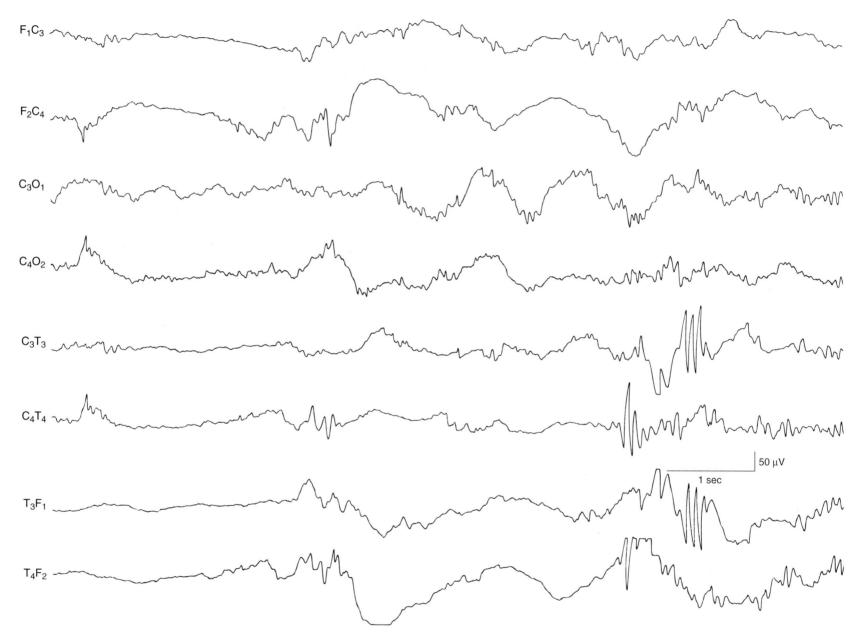

**FIG. 4–12. 33 weeks CA. Bilateral, asynchronous, temporal alpha bursts.** Alpha bursts are present in the temporal regions, appearing independently and asynchronously on the two sides.

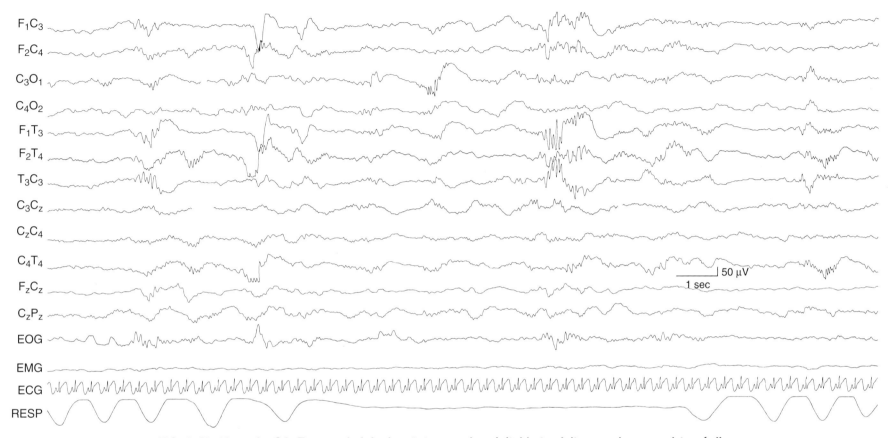

**FIG. 4–13. 33 weeks CA. Temporal alpha burst, temporal occipital beta–delta complexes, and *tracé discontinu*.** Temporal bursts with a frequency in the alpha range are present on the left. Beta–delta complexes are present in the occipital and temporal regions. The background activity is discontinuous, although less so than in recordings of infants of a younger CA.

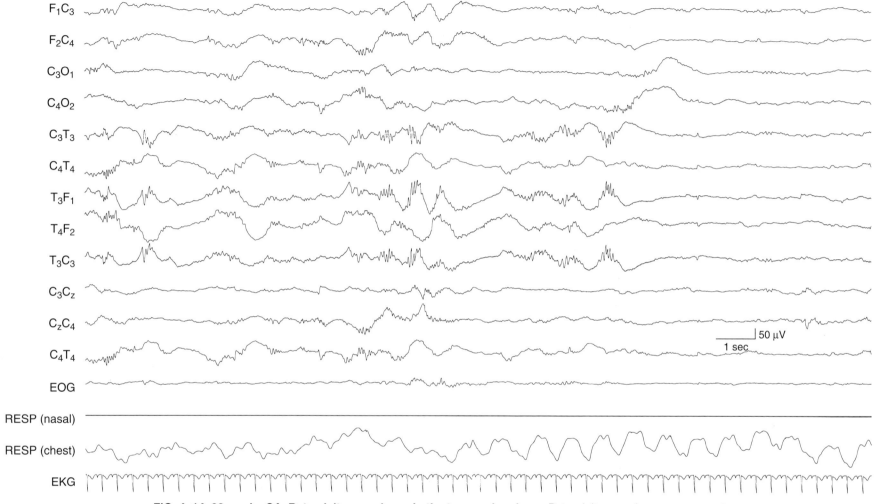

**FIG. 4–14. 33 weeks CA. Beta–delta complexes in the temporal regions.** Beta–delta complexes are present in the temporal regions, greater on the left. A brief run of alpha-frequency activity appears in the left temporal region. The background activity is discontinuous. Periods of discontinuity are shorter, and the periods of bursting activity are longer than those in infants with a younger CA.

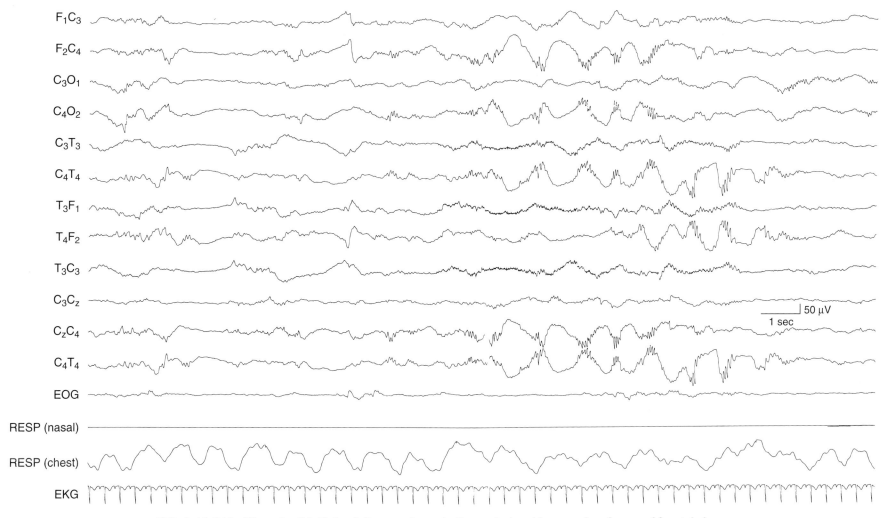

**FIG. 4–15. 34 to 35 weeks CA. Beta–delta complexes in the central and temporal regions and frontal sharp transients.** Beta–delta complexes are present in the right central region followed by beta–delta complexes in the right temporal region. Rudimentary frontal sharp transients, higher in amplitude and more well formed on the right side in the early portion of the sample, suggest that the CA of this infant is early in the 34- to 35-week epoch.

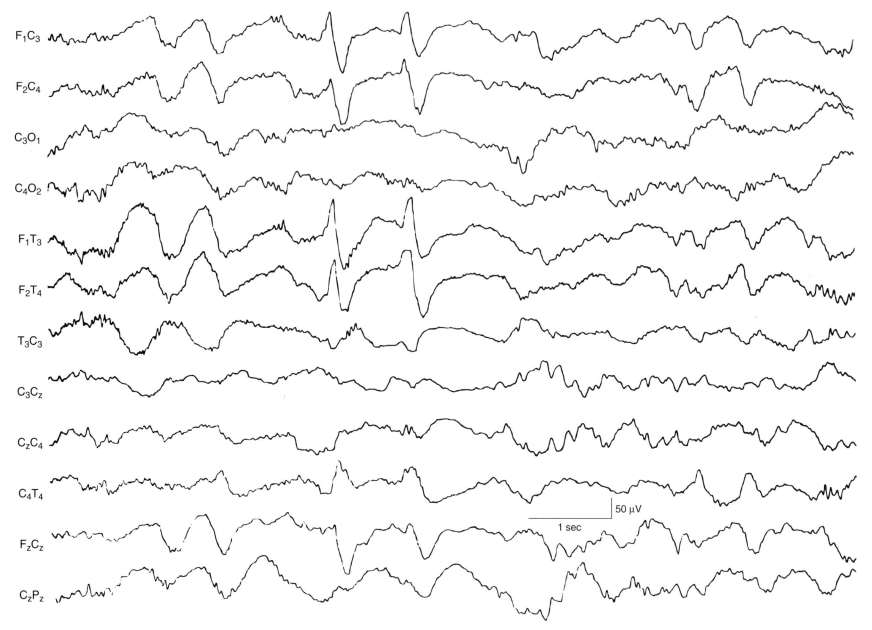

**FIG. 4–16. 34 to 35 weeks CA. Frontal sharp transients.** Bilaterally, synchronous diphasic sharp transients are present in the frontal leads.

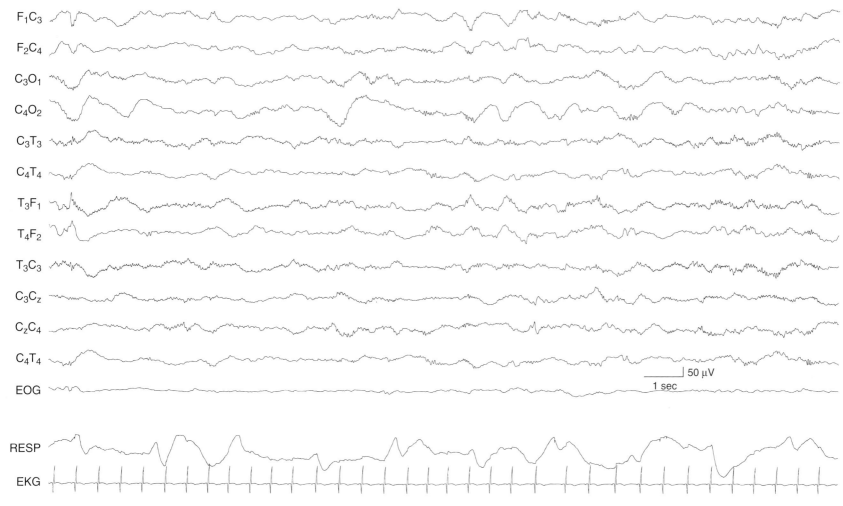

**FIG. 4–17. 34 to 35 weeks CA. Awake: relative continuous background activity with some interhemispheric asynchrony.** The background activity is continuous, with intermittent beta–delta complexes in the occipital regions. This sample is from the same recording of the infant in Fig. 4–18.

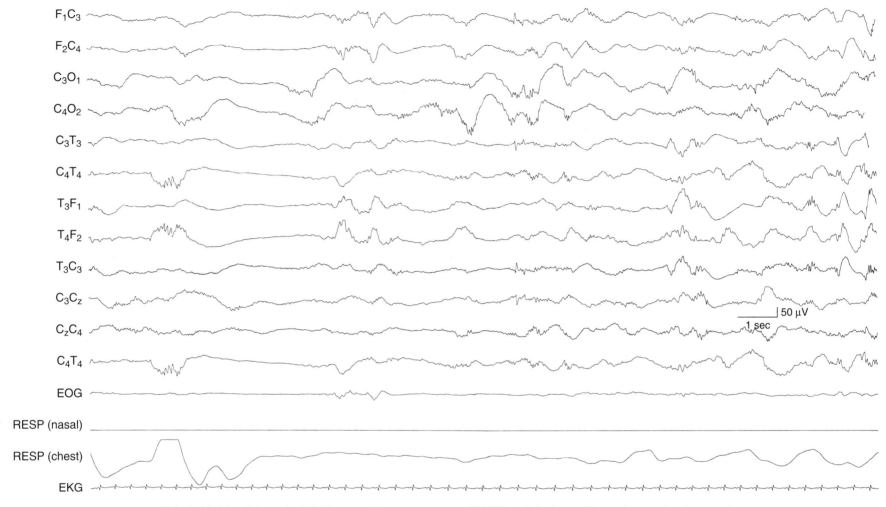

**FIG. 4–18. 34 to 35 weeks CA. Non–rapid eye movement (NREM; quiet) sleep: discontinuous background activity.** A period of discontinuity appears during NREM sleep. This sample is from the same recording of the infant from Fig. 4–17.

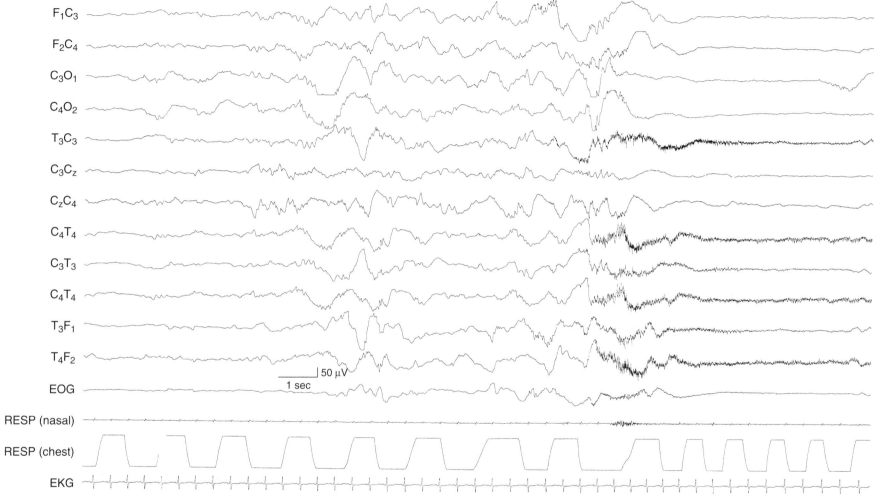

**FIG. 4–19. 36 to 37 weeks CA. Arousal from non–rapid eye movement (NREM; quiet) sleep: generalized voltage attenuation associated with clinical arousal.** The early portion of the sample demonstrates the discontinuity of NREM (quiet) sleep. The infant then self-arouses. This is associated with generalized voltage attenuation (and electromyographic artifact from the temporalis muscles).

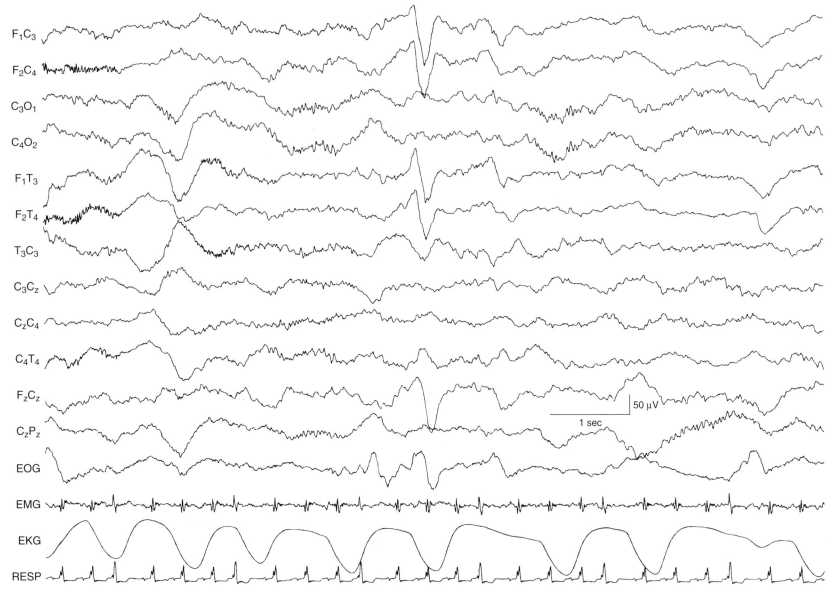

**FIG. 4–20. 36 to 37 weeks CA. Frontal sharp transients, continuous polyfrequency activity, and a paucity of beta–delta complexes.** Frontal sharp transients occur synchronously and symmetrically on the two sides. The background activity is relatively continuous with polyfrequency activity throughout, although there is still beta-complex activity posteriorly.

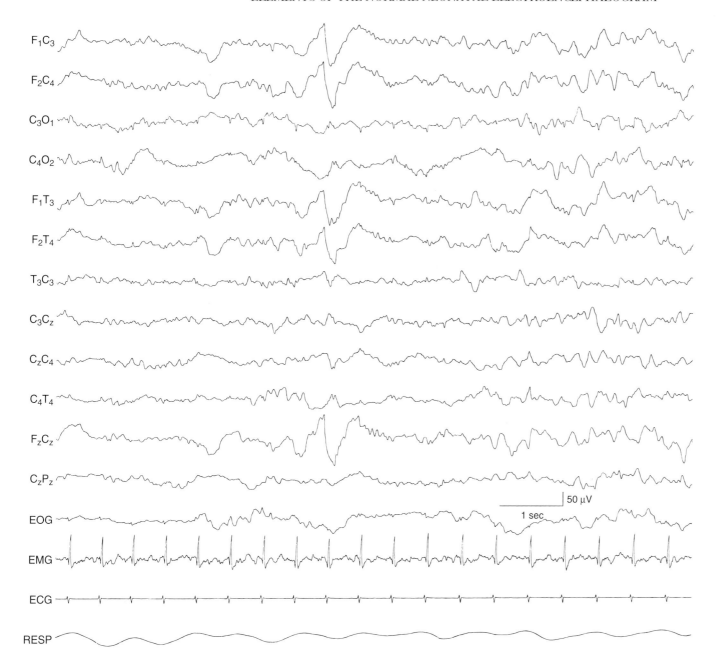

**FIG. 4–21. 38 to 40 weeks CA. Frontal sharp transients with continuous background activity.** Bilateral, synchronous, frontal sharp transients occur randomly. Their occurrence is similar to those of earlier CAs when they first emerge as developmental landmarks, but at this CA, frontal sharp transients occur with continuous background activity.

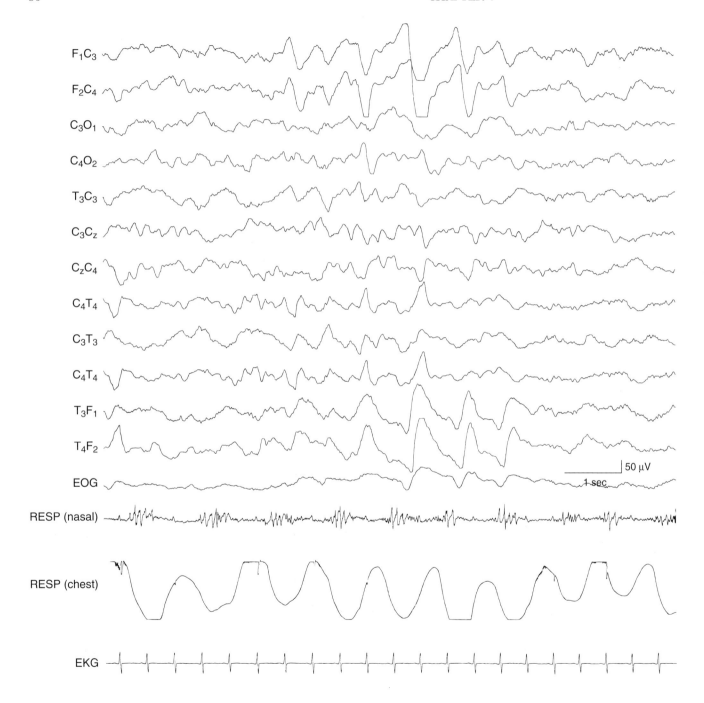

**FIG. 4–22. 38 to 40 weeks CA. Repetitive frontal sharp transients.** As at younger CAs, frontal sharp transients may occur in brief runs.

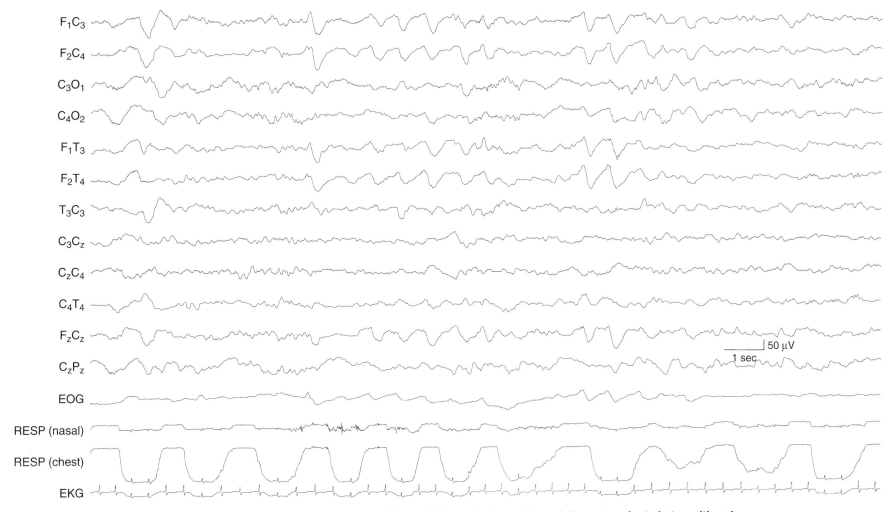

**FIG. 4–23. 38 to 40 weeks CA. Rhythmic bifrontal delta activity and frontal sharp transients in transitional sleep.** Intermittent bifrontal delta activity, at times, is mixed with frontal sharp transients. Bifrontal delta activity is not a developmental landmark, *per se*, but this activity is considered a normal variation typically occurring in transitional or indeterminant sleep. See text for further details to differentiate normal from abnormal bifrontal delta activity.

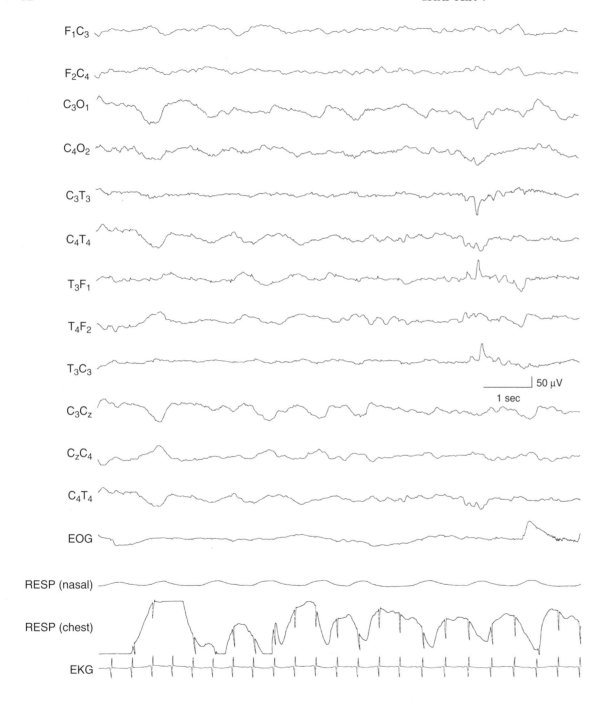

**FIG. 4–24. 38 to 40 weeks CA. Temporal sharp waves.** A moderate-voltage sharp wave in the left temporal region occurs in isolation. The background activity is normal for CA. Randomly occurring, moderate-voltage sharp waves do occur in the EEGs that are otherwise normal and in neonates who also are normal. A continuum of the degree of normality-to-abnormality of these waveforms is discussed in Chapter 5. This sample is presented to indicate that some temporal sharp waves can be considered normal, although the presence of temporal sharp waves does not constitute a developmental landmark.

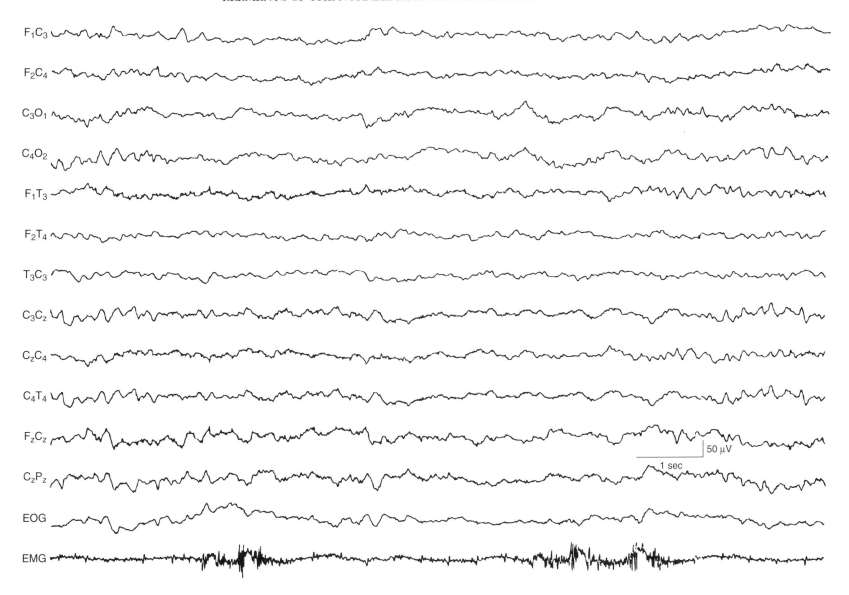

**FIG. 4–25. 38 to 40 weeks CA. Awake: continuous, synchronous polyfrequency activity.** The continuous and synchronous polyfrequency activity includes a mixture of alpha, beta, theta, and delta activity. (From Hrachovy RA. Development of the normal electroencephalogram. In: Levin KH, Luders HO, eds. *Comprehensive clinical neurophysiology.* Philadelphia: WB Saunders, 2000:387–413, with permission.)

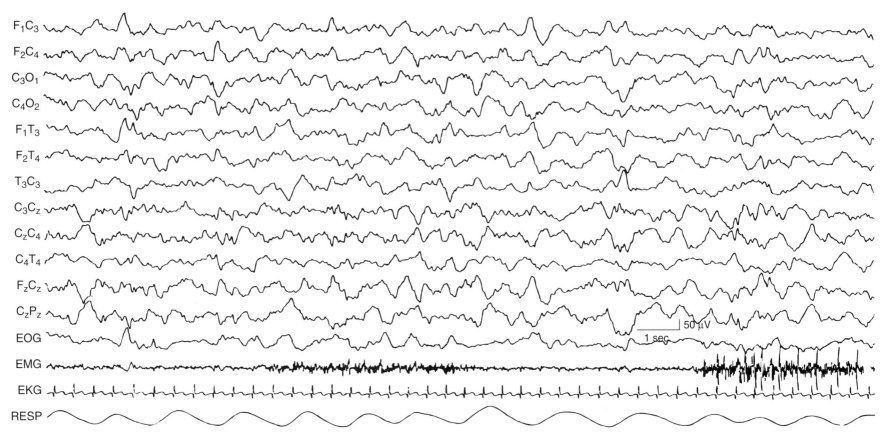

**FIG. 4–26. 38 to 40 weeks CA. Non–rapid eye movement (REM; quiet) sleep: continuous slow activity.**
Continuous, relatively slow activity is synchronous on the two sides. Respiration is regular, and no REMs occur. (From Hrachovy RA. Development of the normal electroencephalogram. In: Levin KH, Luders HO, eds. *Comprehensive clinical neurophysiology.* Philadelphia: WB Saunders, 2000:387–413, with permission.)

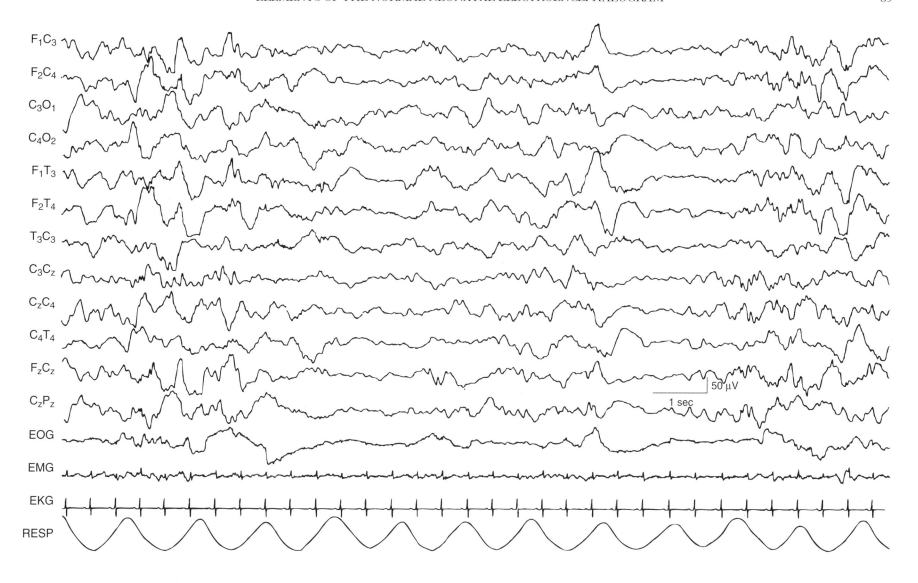

**FIG. 4–27. 38 to 40 weeks CA.** *Tracé alternant* **in deep non–rapid eye movement (NREM; quiet) sleep.** Periods of discontinuity occur during periods of deep NREM. (From Hrachovy RA. Development of the normal electroencephalogram. In: Levin KH, Luders HO, eds. *Comprehensive clinical neurophysiology.* Philadelphia: WB Saunders, 2000:387–413, with permission.)

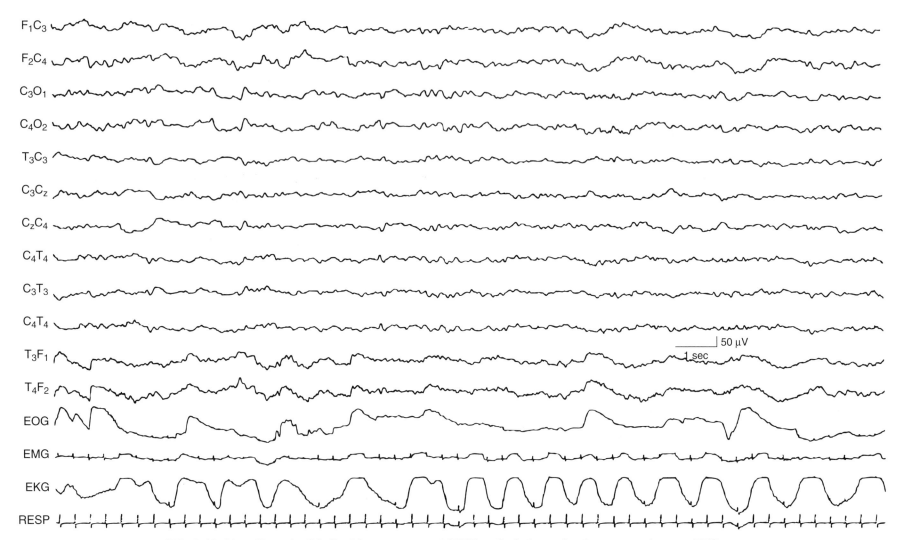

**FIG. 4–28. 38 to 40 weeks CA. Rapid eye movement (REM; active) sleep.** Continuous, synchronous EEG activity occurs. Respiration is irregular, and REMs are recorded on the electrooculogram channel. (From Hrachovy RA. Development of the normal electroencephalogram. In: Levin KH, Luders HO, eds. *Comprehensive clinical neurophysiology.* Philadelphia: WB Saunders, 2000:387–413, with permission.)

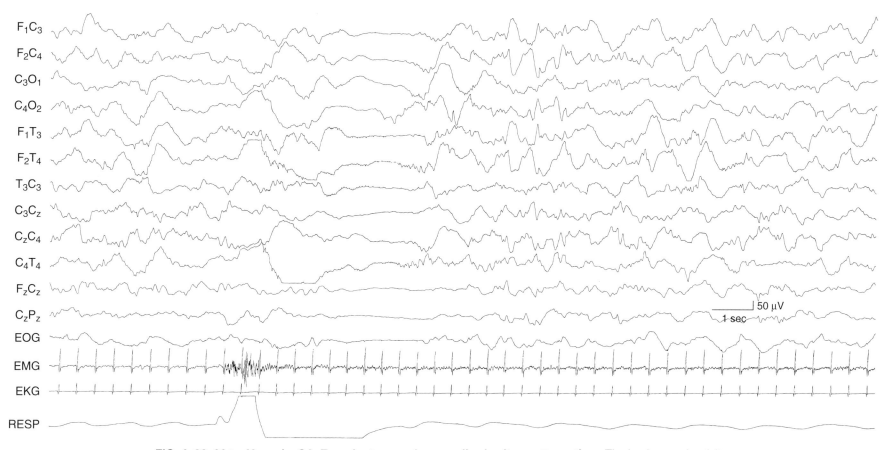

**FIG. 4–29. 38 to 40 weeks CA. Transient arousal: generalized voltage attenuation.** The background activity is consistent with non–rapid eye movement (NREM; quiet) sleep. A brief episode of generalized voltage attenuation is associated with clinical arousal (the electromyogram and respiration channels indicate movement). After about 2 seconds, the EEG returns to NREM background.

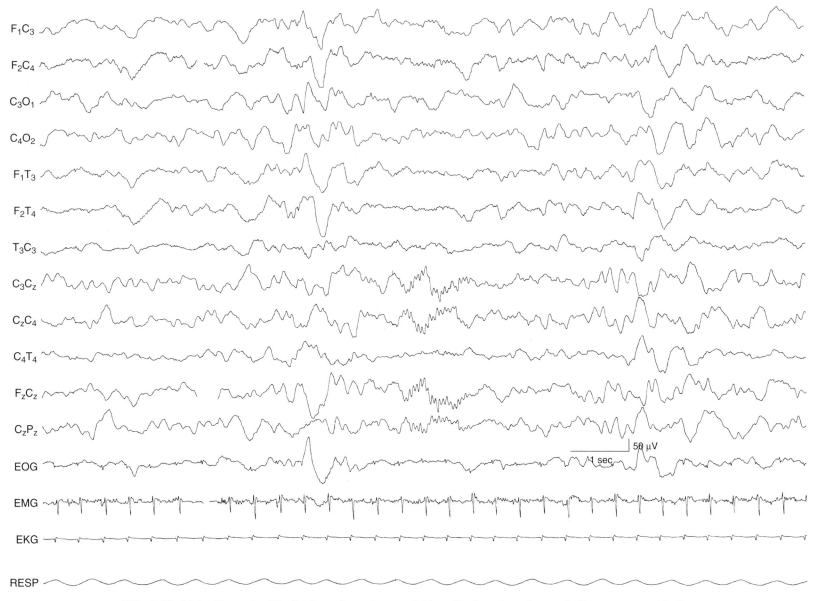

**FIG. 4–30. 41 to 44 weeks CA. Rudimentary sleep spindles.** Rudimentary sleep spindles are present in the midline central region in this 43-week CA infant during non–rapid eye movement (NREM; quiet) sleep. The background activity is continuous. This is not a typical finding in this CA epoch because spindles are most consistently present after 6 weeks post-term. However, on rare occasions, rudimentary spindles occur earlier, and when they first appear are present in the midline central region as shown.

**FIGURES CONTINUE ON THE NEXT PAGE**

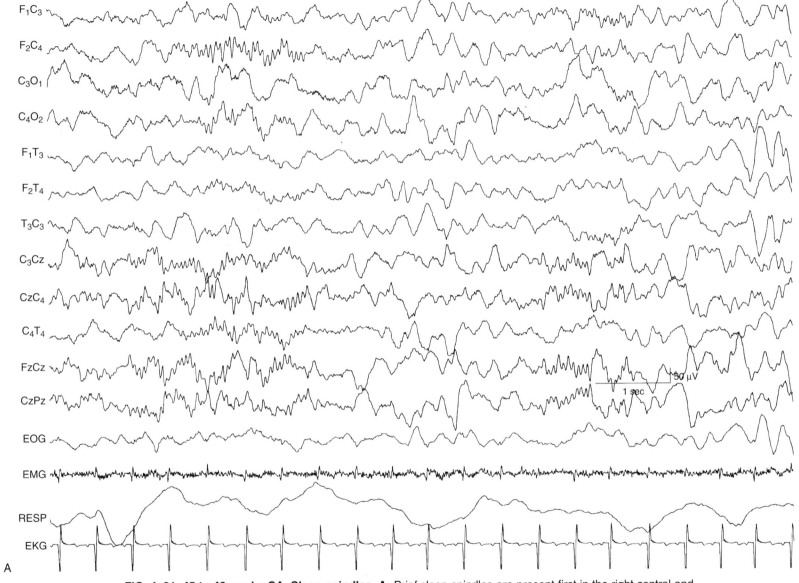

F₁C₃
F₂C₄
C₃O₁
C₄O₂
F₁T₃
F₂T₄
T₃C₃
C₃Cz
CzC₄
C₄T₄
FzCz
CzPz
EOG
EMG
RESP
EKG

50 μV

1 sec

A

**FIG. 4–31. 45 to 48 weeks CA. Sleep spindles. A:** Brief sleep spindles are present first in the right central and then in the left central regions in the EEG of this 46-week CA infant. Both bursts have some midline central localization. **B:** This sample is a continuation of the sample shown in **A.** Now the spindles are longer, with those on the right beginning first, overlapping in time with that on the left. The spindles on the two sides occur simultaneously for a few seconds, and then the spindle on the right subsides while that on the left persists for several seconds.

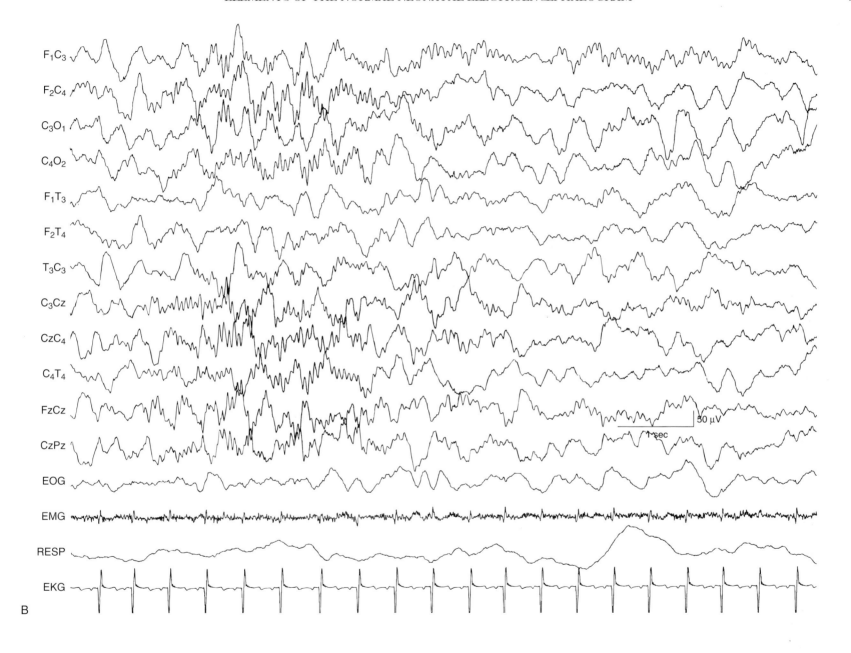

B

# CHAPTER 5

# Patterns of Uncertain Diagnostic Significance

A number of waveforms and patterns have not been reported to occur in normal infants, do not fit criteria of normality, and are not associated with well-defined abnormal clinical correlates. These patterns are of questionable or uncertain diagnostic significance.

## FOCAL SHARP WAVES

Currently, little understanding exists of the significance of focal sharp waves in premature and term infants. Various definitions of "normal" spikes and sharp waves have been proposed. For example, spikes or sharp waves occurring two or three times in an hour-long recording have no significance in the newborn. To be considered normal, spikes and sharp waves occurring more frequently than this must be truly random and without persistent focality (Monod et al., 1972) and may arise from any scalp location (Engel, 1975; Hagne, 1972; Schulte, 1970). However, no stringent criteria have been developed to separate, unambiguously, abnormal from normal sharp-wave activity in the newborn.

Sharp waves or sharp-and-slow-wave complexes are commonly recorded from the midtemporal region during sleep in apparently normal premature and term infants. The features our group uses to differentiate between normal and abnormal temporal sharp waves are as follows:

### Amplitude and Duration

In general, as the amplitude and duration of sharp waves increase, so does the likelihood that they are abnormal. For example, in a premature or term infant, random midtemporal sharp waves having a voltage of less than 75 μV, a duration of less than 100 milliseconds, and occurring only rarely during sleep would be consid-

ered normal (**Fig. 5–1**). Conversely, midtemporal sharp waves with a voltage exceeding 150 μV and a duration greater than 150 milliseconds would be considered abnormal. Unfortunately, numerous temporal sharp waves fall in a "gray zone" between these criteria. The most controversial is that of amplitude, because some sharp waves of greater than 100 μV may be considered normal if they are normal by all other parameters. However, other features, discussed in this section, often aid the neurophysiologist in determining the probability of normality or abnormality.

### Incidence and Persistence

Temporal sharp waves that are considered normal occur randomly. They usually occur bilaterally but asynchronously and may be symmetrical or asymmetrical (**Fig. 5–2**). Generally these sharp waves appear infrequently; thus temporal sharp waves occurring in quick succession or long runs and sharp waves occurring on only one side are more likely to be considered abnormal (**Figs. 5–3 to 5–5**).

### Morphology and Complexity of Waveforms

Temporal sharp waves classified as normal are usually mono- or diphasic. The morphology of abnormal temporal sharp waves is more variable. Although they are sometimes mono- or diphasic, abnormal sharp waves more often are polyphasic and followed by an extremely high voltage slow wave (**Figs. 5–6 to 5–9**).

### Polarity

The initial component of a normal temporal sharp wave is surface negative. Temporal sharp waves with an initial or prominent surface-positive component are abnormal (**Fig. 5–9**).

## Features Associated with Changes in Wake/Sleep States

In the premature infant, normal temporal sharp waves occur in any state. In the term infant, however, normal temporal sharp waves are more common during transitional sleep. If temporal sharp waves appear in the waking record of term infants, they probably are abnormal, regardless of other characteristics (**Fig. 5–10**). Midtemporal sharp waves satisfying the above criteria of normality occur in some healthy term newborns during sleep. These sharp waves disappear rapidly during the first month of life and are seen in fewer than 5% of healthy newborns after 6 weeks postterm. Even temporal sharp waves considered clearly abnormal often do not persist beyond this age.

## FOCAL RHYTHMIC ACTIVITY

### Midline Frontal Rhythmic Theta and Alpha Activity

Bursts of rhythmic 50- to 200-$\mu$V, 5- to 9-Hz activity may occur in the midline frontal regions of neurologically normal infants between 38 and 42 weeks CA (Hayakawa et al., 1987). The waves may have a sharp appearance, may occur in brief bursts usually lasting less than 1.5 seconds, and may occur in transitional or non–rapid eye movement (NREM) sleep, although typically not in REM sleep. They have been reported to occur in 55% of neurologically normal term infants, only rarely occur in infants with abnormal outcomes (4% of abnormal infants), and are not present in infants with moderate to severely depressed background activity (Hayakawa et al., 1987).

### Midline Central Rhythmic Theta and Alpha Activity

Rhythmic activity similar to the frontal midline activity described earlier also may be present in the midline central region in an otherwise normal EEG (Hrachovy et al., 1990) (**Figs. 5–11 to 5–13**). This activity also may accompany other EEG features that are considered abnormal, particularly central sharp waves, in infants who have experienced various central nervous system (CNS) insults.

### Occipital Rhythmic Theta Activity

In the term infant's EEG, an uncommon finding is the occurrence of brief runs of rhythmic 4- to 6-Hz, 50- to 100-$\mu$V activity in the occipital regions with a duration of less than 1 second. This activity appears in wakefulness or sleep and usually occurs asynchronously on the two sides. In some infants, this activity may be unilateral. Occipital rhythmic theta activity can occur as an isolated feature in an otherwise normal EEG, but usually it accompanies other abnormalities such as sharp waves or an abnormal background (**Fig. 5–14**).

## TRANSIENT UNILATERAL ATTENUATION OF BACKGROUND ACTIVITY DURING SLEEP

Transient unilateral attenuation of background EEG activity occurring during slow-wave sleep is an unusual finding reported to occur in about 3% to 4% of all newborns (Challamal et al., 1984; O'Brien et al., 1987) (**Fig. 5–15**). The attenuation episodes usually last about 1 minute and begin and end abruptly. The background EEG activity is normal in many infants. In our experience, these episodes usually occur only once during a recording session and usually within minutes of the time the infant first enters NREM sleep.

The significance of this finding, which occurs in apparently normal as well as in abnormal infants, has not been determined. Such episodes of unilateral attenuation of background activity should not be confused with the more common finding of marked generalized and/or lateralized voltage attenuation seen in the EEGs of infants who have experienced a variety of CNS insults. The latter attenuation episodes are short in duration (2–15 seconds), occur repeatedly during the recording session, and may be present in all states. The isolated transient unilateral attenuation episodes seen in slow-wave sleep and the generalized and/or lateralized attenuation episodes associated with various CNS insults also must be distinguished from the generalized attenuation of background EEG activity that is seen when transient arousal occurs during NREM sleep.

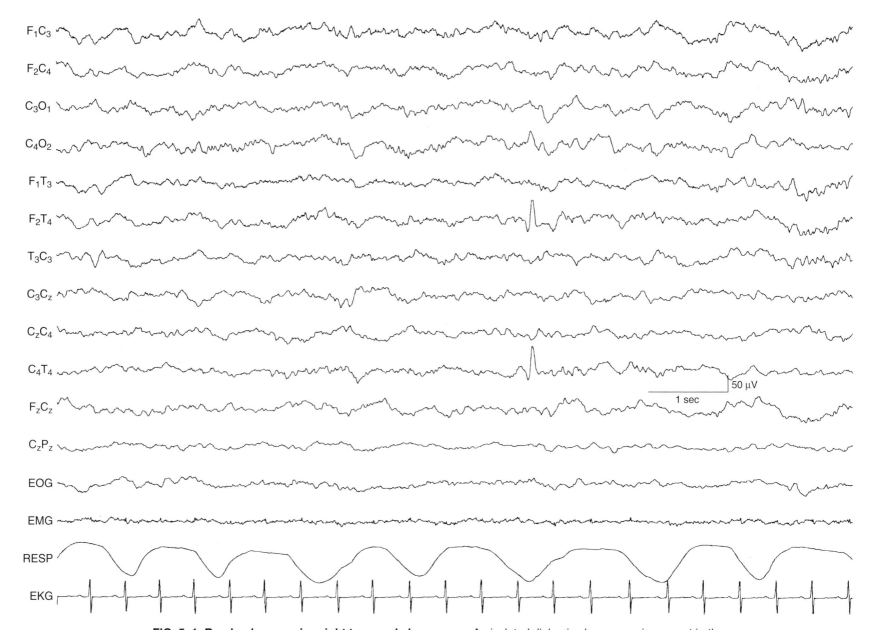

**FIG. 5–1. Randomly occurring right temporal sharp wave.** An isolated diphasic sharp wave is present in the right temporal region with features that suggest it is a normal phenomenon. The background EEG of this sleeping 40-week CA infant is normal.

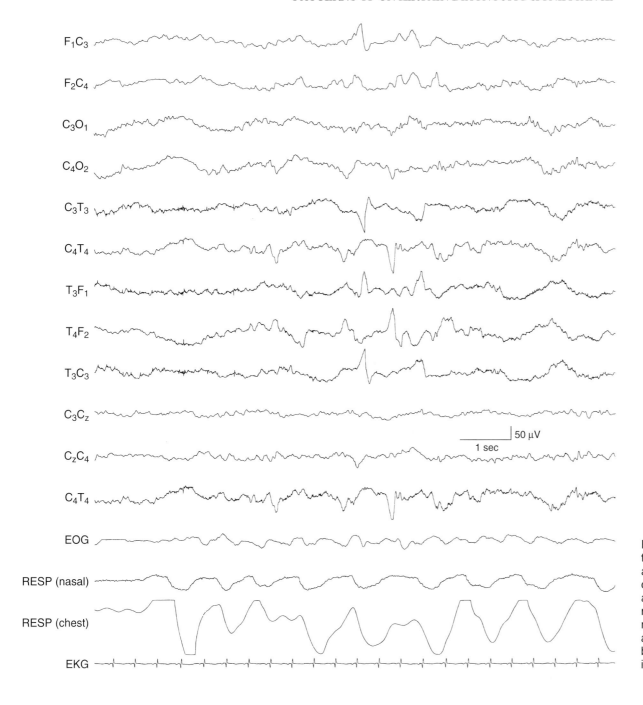

**FIG. 5–2. Independent, symmetrical, bilateral temporal sharp waves.** Sharp waves in the left and right temporal regions appear asynchronously, but symmetrically. The bilateral and asynchronous nature of the sharp waves is a normal finding. However, their amplitudes are near or greater than 150 μV, and their duration are relatively long, suggesting abnormality. The background activity is normal in this 40-week CA infant.

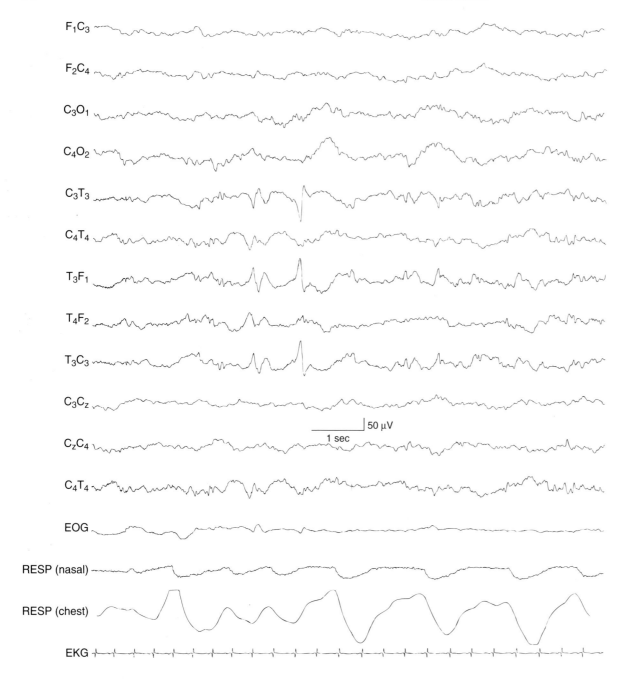

F₁C₃

F₂C₄

C₃O₁

C₄O₂

C₃T₃

C₄T₄

T₃F₁

T₄F₂

T₃C₃

C₃Cz

| 50 μV
___ 1 sec

CzC₄

C₄T₄

EOG

RESP (nasal)

RESP (chest)

EKG

**FIG. 5–3. Repetitive left temporal sharp waves.** Recurring sharp waves are present in the left temporal region in this 40-week CA infant with normal EEG background activity. Only two sharp waves are present in this sample; thus, although repetitive, the degree of repetition is marginal. Additional sharp waves occurring in the recording would have to be analyzed before making a final determination of normality.

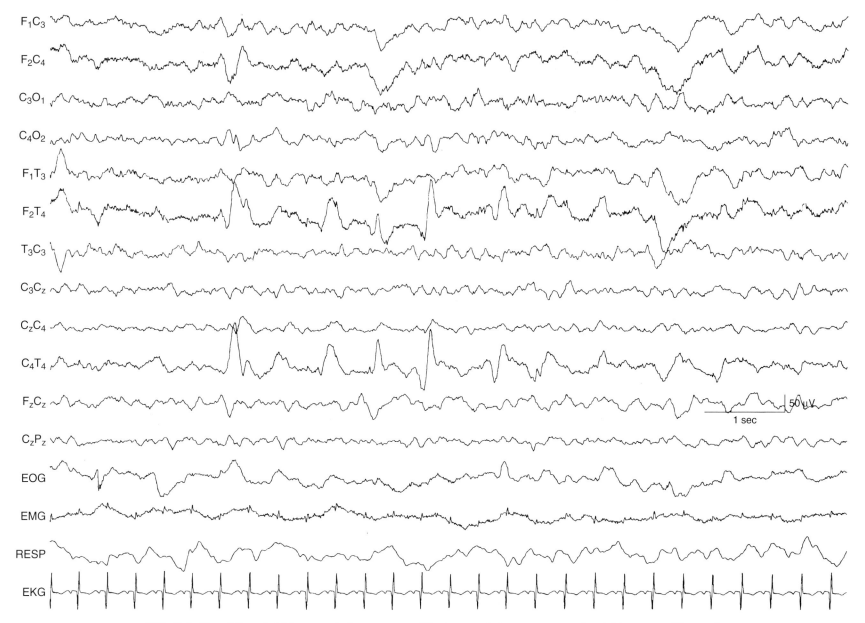

**FIG. 5–4. Repetitive right temporal sharp waves.** The temporal sharp waves on the right are repetitive and high in amplitude. These features suggest abnormality. The background EEG activity is normal in this 40-week CA infant (low-frequency filter, 1.0 Hz).

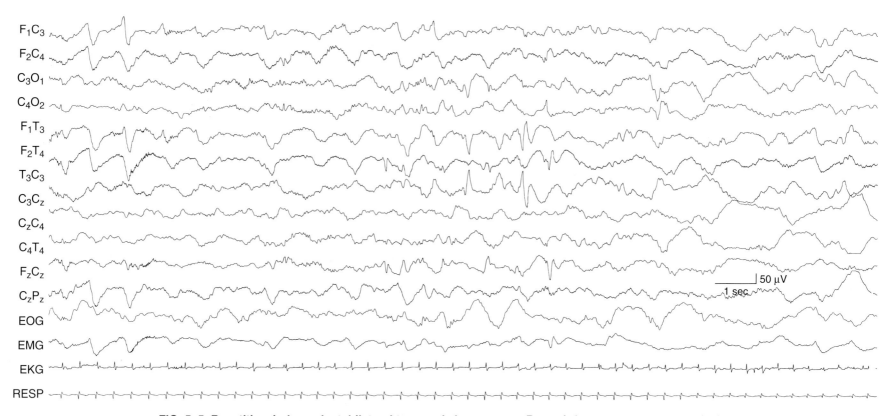

**FIG. 5–5. Repetitive, independent, bilateral temporal sharp waves.** Runs of sharp waves are present in the left and right temporal regions, more prominently on the left where the sharp waves are more frequent and higher in amplitude than those on the right. The repetitive occurrence and the high amplitude of some of the waves and their association with slow waves on the left suggest abnormality. Note the frontal sharp transients in the early portion of the sample; their occurrence is a normal phenomenon at this CA. This sleeping infant is 40 weeks CA, and normal background EEG activity is present.

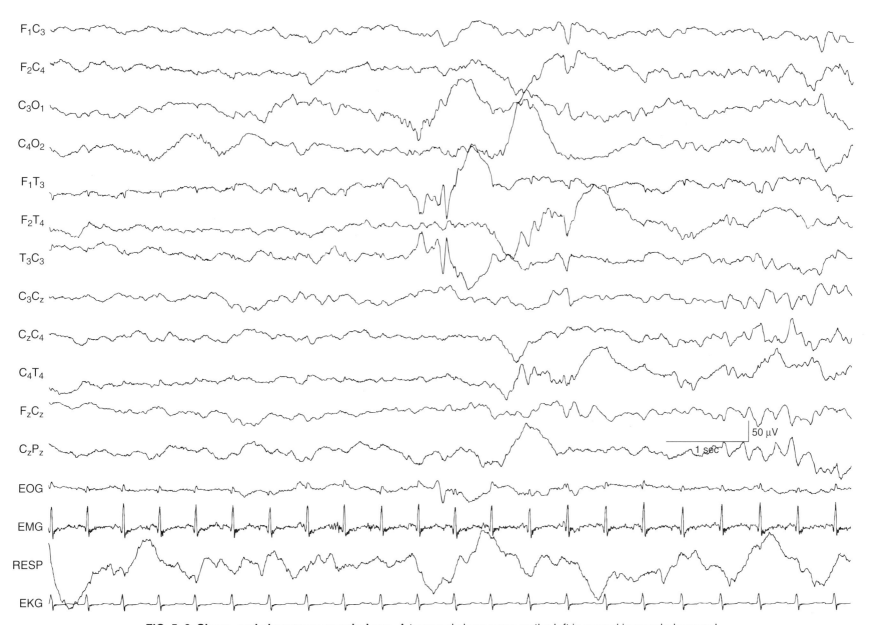

**FIG. 5–6. Sharp- and slow-wave morphology.** A temporal sharp wave on the left is normal in morphology and marginal in amplitude. However, the high-voltage slow wave that follows the sharp wave (creating a sharp- and slow-wave complex) suggests that this is an abnormal finding. This 42-week CA infant is in non–rapid eye movement (quiet) sleep. The background activity is normal.

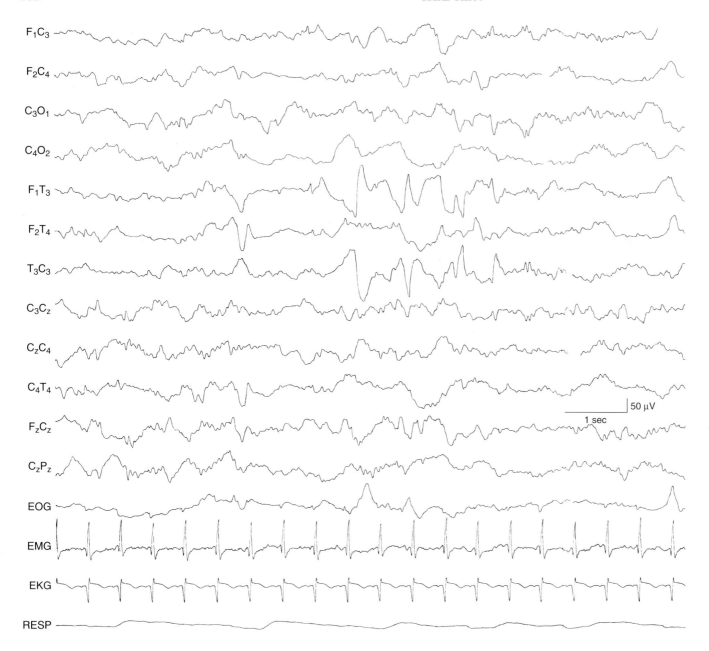

**FIG. 5–7. Complex morphology of left temporal sharp waves.** The morphology of the sharp-wave activity in the left temporal region is relatively complex, with slow and fast components and some waveforms that are sharper than others, suggesting abnormality. The background EEG activity is normal in this 38-week CA infant.

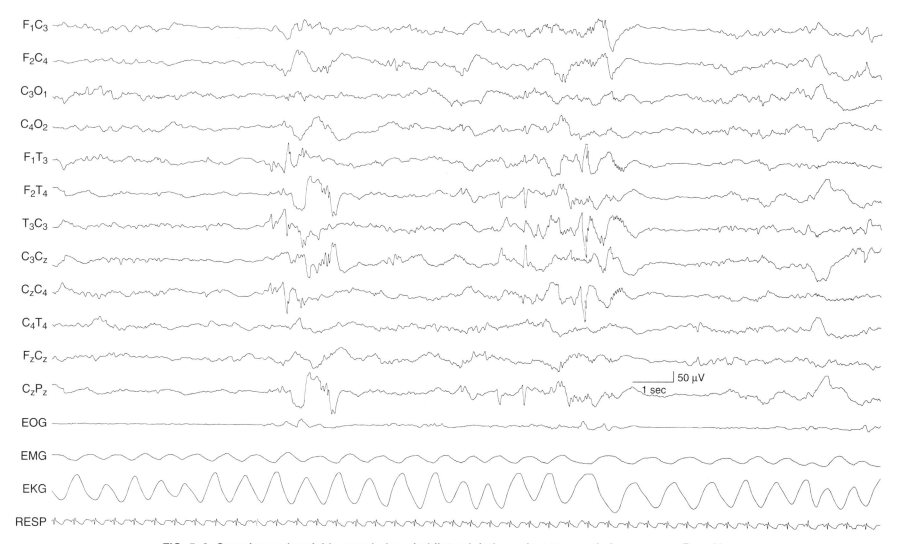

**FIG. 5–8. Complex and variable morphology in bilateral, independent temporal sharp waves.** Repetitive temporal sharp waves appear independently in the left and right temporal regions with complex morphology, including spike-like waveforms. These features suggest that these temporal sharp waves are abnormal. The background EEG activity is abnormal with brief episodes of generalized voltage attenuation in this 40-week CA infant.

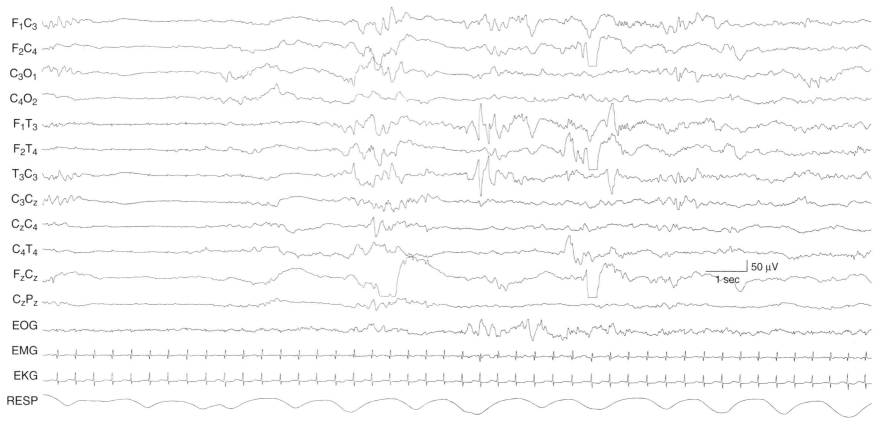

**FIG. 5–9. Complex morphology and varying polarity of temporal sharp waves.** The sharp wave activity appears independently in the left and right temporal regions. Variable and complex morphology is present in both regions, with waveform components that are both surface negative and surface positive in polarity. The EEG background is abnormal, with brief periods of voltage attenuation in this 40-week CA infant.

**FIGURES CONTINUE ON THE NEXT PAGE**

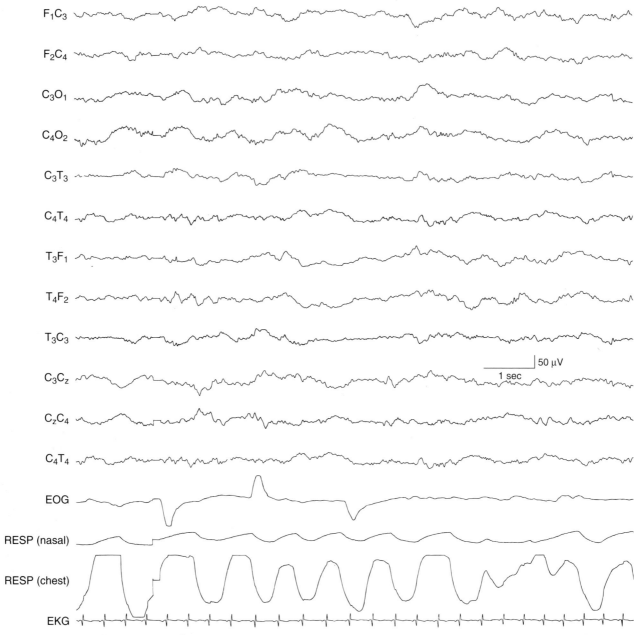

**FIG. 5–10. Influence of wake/sleep state on the occurrence of temporal sharp waves: activation of sharp waves during sleep. A:** The awake recording in this 40-week CA infant is normal with continuous polyfrequency activity and no sharp waves. *(continued)*

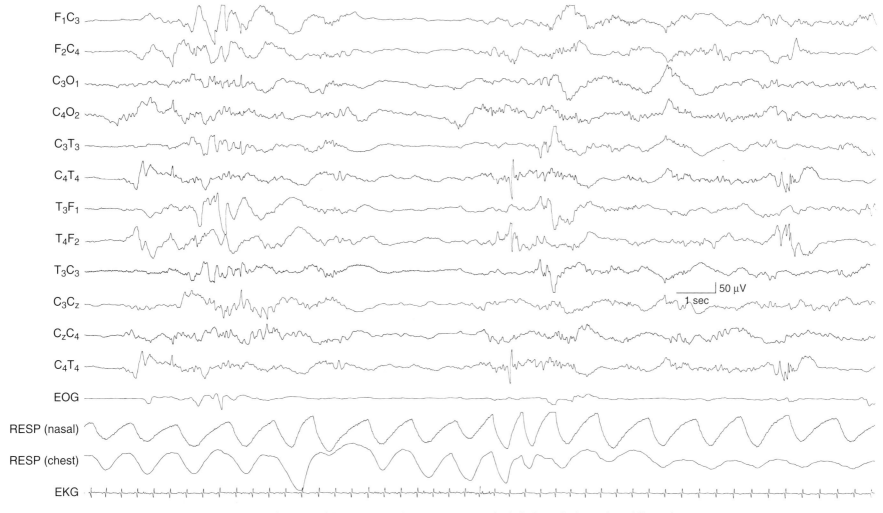

**FIG. 5–10.** *(Continued)* **B:** In non–rapid eye movement (quiet) sleep, independent, bilateral temporal sharp waves are found with variable and complex morphology. The background activity is characterized by abnormal periods of generalized voltage attenuation. This recording is from the same infant shown in Fig. 5–9.

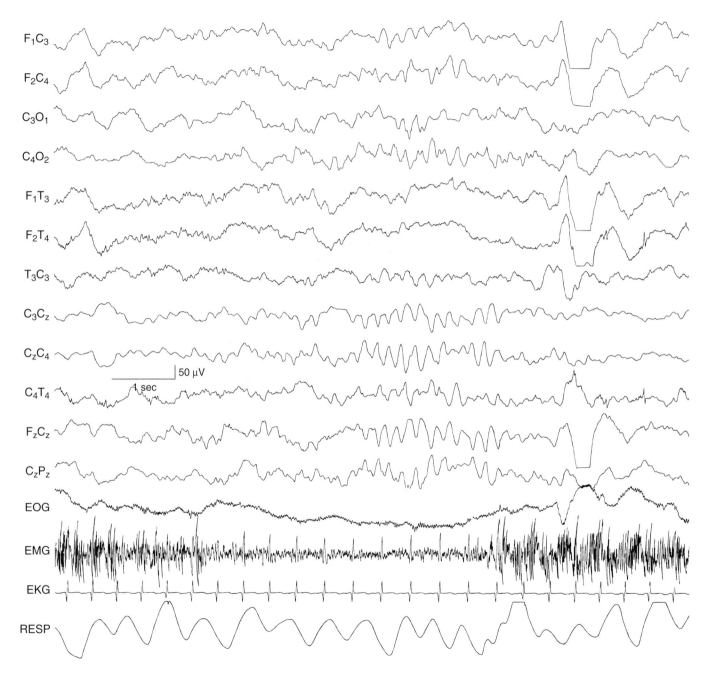

**FIG. 5–11. Brief burst of rhythmic theta activity in the midline central region.** A brief burst of rhythmic theta activity is seen in the midline central (Cz) region in this sample from a 40-week CA infant with normal background EEG activity.

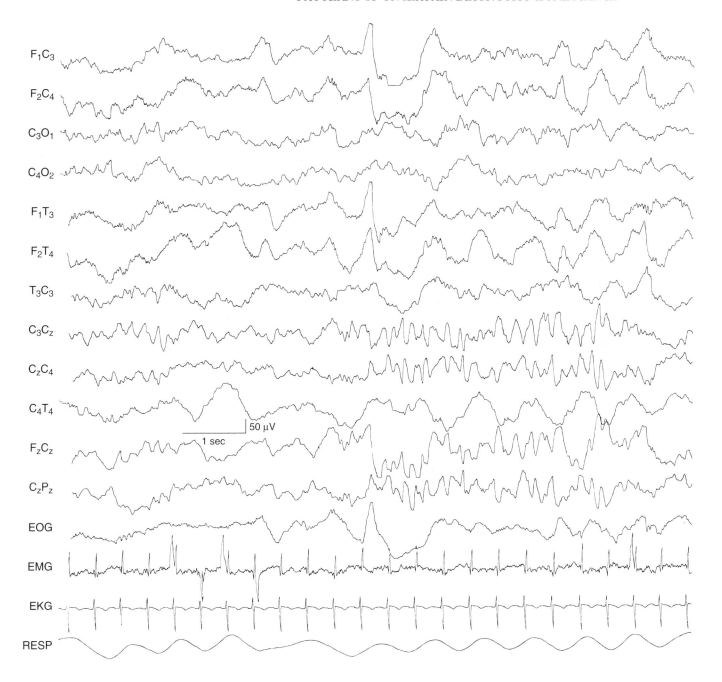

**FIG. 5–12. Sustained burst of rhythmic theta activity in the midline central region.** A sustained burst of rhythmic theta activity is present in the midline central (Cz) region. Normal frontal sharp transients are present. The background EEG activity is normal in this 40-week CA infant.

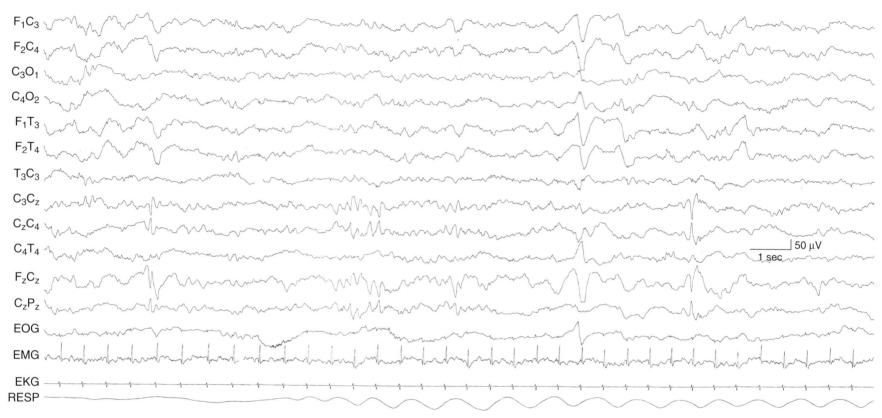

**FIG. 5–13. Rhythmic midline central theta bursts and midline central sharp waves.** A brief run of rhythmic theta activity occurs in the midline central region in the middle portion of this sample. Earlier and later, sharp waves or spikes in the same region are more abnormal features. Frontal sharp transients, normal waveforms, are present, and the EEG background activity is normal in this 40-week CA infant.

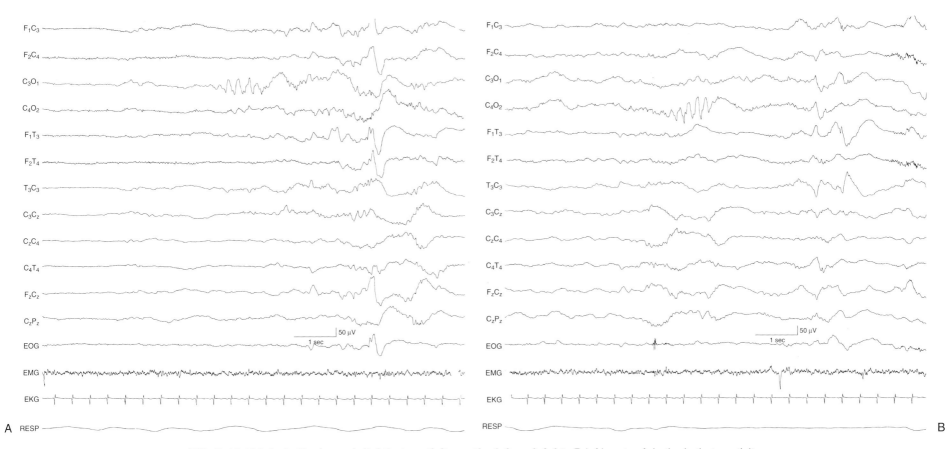

**FIG. 5–14. Brief, rhythmic occipital theta activity on the left and right.** Brief bursts of rhythmic theta activity in the left **(A)** and right **(B)** occipital regions appear on two samples from one EEG recording in this 34-week CA infant.

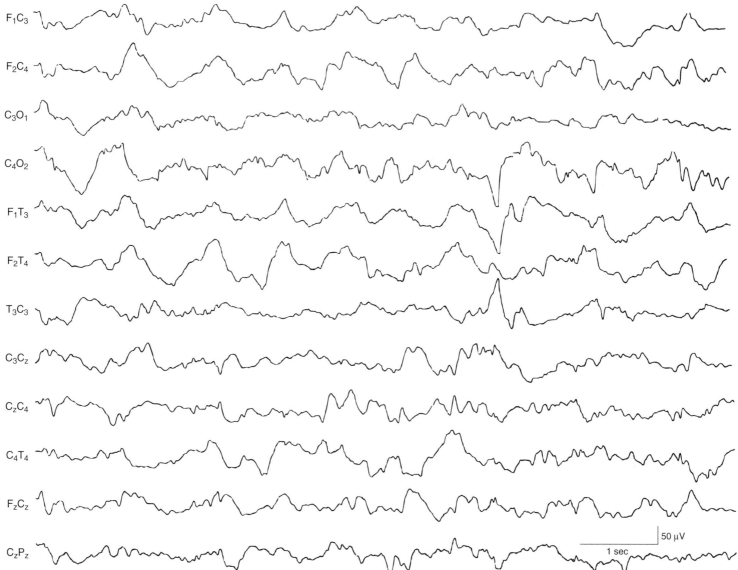

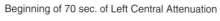

**FIG. 5–15. Transient unilateral attenuation of background activity during sleep.** Selected segments are shown of an episode of transient unilateral attenuation of background activity during sleep, lasting 70 seconds. **A:** Initially voltage attenuation of activity occurs in leads from the left hemisphere. *(continued)*

Middle of Attenuation

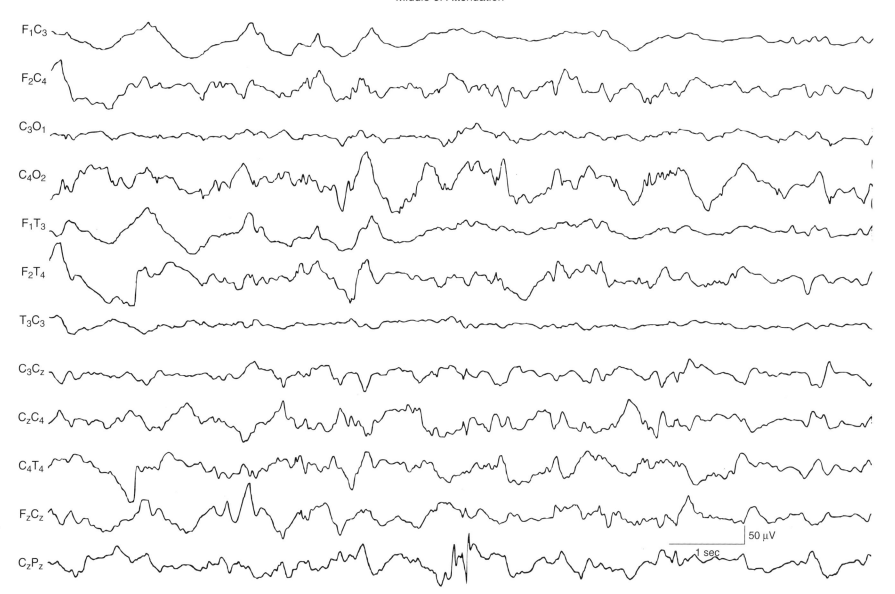

**FIG. 5–15.** *(Continued)* **B:** The attenuation persists for several seconds. *(continued)*

End of Attenuation

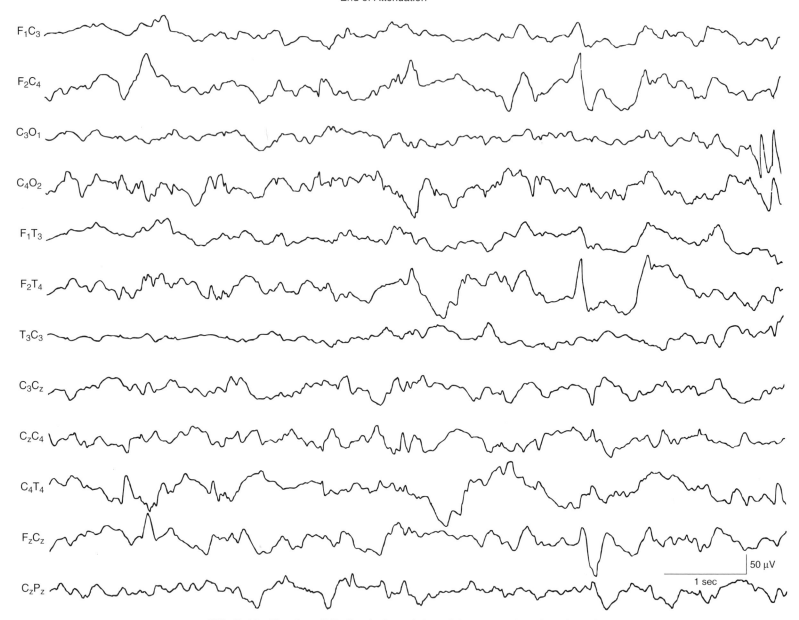

**FIG. 5–15.** *(Continued)* **C:** Gradual resolution of the attenuation. *(continued)*

Post attenuation

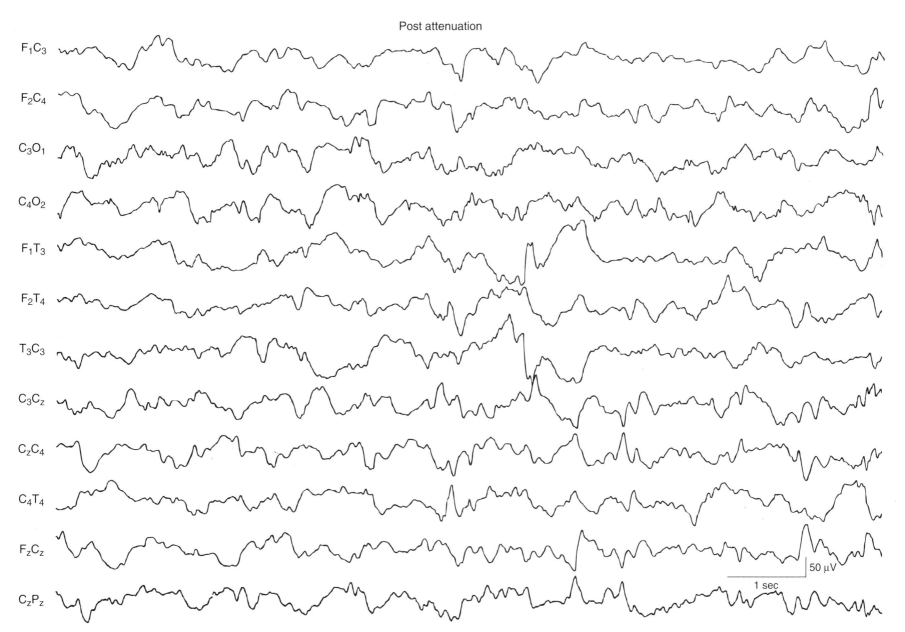

**FIG. 5–15.** *(Continued)* **D:** The EEG eventually returns to baseline. The background EEG activity is normal in this 40-week CA infant.

# Electroencephalographic Abnormalities of Premature and Term Neonates

## TIMING OF ELECTROENCEPHALOGRAPHIC STUDIES

Ideally, the initial electroencephalogram (EEG) examination should be done within the first 24 hours after birth or after a suspected brain insult. The best estimate of the degree of damage or dysfunction can be made when the EEG documents the evolution of the abnormality over time. Typically, as time passes, the degree of abnormality lessens. The slower this change, the more severe the underlying brain abnormality. If serial studies document the rate and character of changes, the prognostic information will be more reliable than that obtained from a single study (Chequer et al., 1992; Douglass et al., 2002; Graziani et al., 1994; Holmes and Lombroso, 1993; Holmes et al., 1982; Klinger et al., 2001; Kumar et al., 1999; Selton and Andre, 1997; Takeuchi and Watanabe, 1989; Tharp et al., 1981; Tharp et al., 1989; Watanabe et al., 1999; Zeinstra et al., 2001). Serial studies also afford greater opportunity to detect electrical seizures (Glauser and Clancy, 1992), the presence of which may be of prognostic significance (see Chapter 7).

Failure to recognize that EEG findings evolve over time may lead to a less than accurate determination of prognosis. For example, an EEG of an infant might show a suppression-burst pattern on the first day after birth, a finding generally indicating the presence of severe brain dysfunction. However, hours later, after the infant's physiological condition has stabilized, the EEG activity may become continuous, with relatively normal background activity. Such changes drastically alter statements concerning the prognosis. On the other hand, a suppression-burst pattern that is sustained over several days or that changes to a depressed and undifferentiated pattern implies a poor prognosis for recovery of brain function. Fail-

ure to recognize the importance of the time course has led to contradictory statements in the literature concerning the prognostic significance of suppression-burst activity.

With this caveat, however, some statements can be made concerning the significance of the first EEG recorded early in the course of neurologic illness. In infants requiring intensive care, the EEG findings obtained within the first 24 hours after birth can provide reliable prognostic information (Pezzani et al., 1986); a normal EEG on the first day, or one with only minimally abnormal findings, reliably indicates a good prognosis unless further brain injury occurs later.

## DIFFUSE ABNORMALITIES

### Dyschronism: Disordered Maturational Development

An experienced neurophysiologist can usually determine CA to within 2 weeks between 27 and 33 weeks CA, and within ±1 week between 34 and 37 weeks CA, based on expected developmental features (see Chapter 4) (Tharp, 1990). Disordered maturational development is referred to as "dyschronism" and, if present, is an important abnormality of the neonatal EEG (Hrachovy et al., 1990).

### *External Dyschronism*

This term refers to an EEG in which the developmental characteristics in all states of sleep and wakefulness are immature for the reported gestational or CA. If the developmental features of an EEG are immature for the stated gestational or CA and the features of the background activity in all states are normal, the following questions must be addressed: (a) Is the age as determined by clinical evaluation overestimated? or (b) Are the immature EEG features evidence of delayed maturation? The latter explanation suggests that a cerebral insult may have occurred during intrauterine life. A discrepancy of 2 weeks or less between EEG age and estimated CA most likely indicates the presence of a transient central nervous system (CNS) dysfunction. However, discrepancies of more than 3 weeks usually indicate persistent impairment of CNS function and are frequently accompanied by other EEG abnormalities, including marked suppression of background activity or multifocal sharp waves.

### Internal Dyschronism

This term refers to different maturational characteristics between the EEG awake and in the deepest stages of non–rapid eye movement (NREM) sleep (**Fig. 6–1**). For example, characteristics of the waking EEG might be consistent with a CA of 38 weeks, whereas the background activity during deep NREM sleep might be consistent with a CA of 34 weeks. If a dyschronism of 3 or more weeks occurs between the awake record and deep sleep, other EEG abnormalities are often present. These abnormalities are usually most apparent in NREM sleep, the state that always shows the least mature characteristics (**Fig. 6–2**). Such findings suggest significant brain dysfunction. Therefore, an EEG of any infant should include a period of the deepest stages of NREM sleep.

### Transient Maturational Abnormalities

Maturational abnormalities may occur transiently in a newborn with acute or ongoing hypoxia–ischemia. Immature EEG characteristics can disappear rapidly when the patient is well oxygenated and the period of hypoxia–ischemia has been short. Therefore, the prognostic significance of an EEG whose developmental features are immature for the stated CA can be determined only by making serial recordings.

## Abnormalities of Background Activity in Diffuse Brain Disturbance

### Prolongation of Interburst Intervals in Premature Infants

The range of the duration of normal interburst intervals is CA dependent and, in older premature infants, state dependent (**Fig. 6–3**). The longest acceptable single interburst interval duration according to CA has been reported to be 26 weeks CA,

46 seconds; 27 weeks, 36 seconds (Selton et al., 2000); less than 30 weeks CA, 30 to 35 seconds; 31 to 33 weeks CA, 20 seconds; 34 to 36 weeks CA, 10 seconds; 37 to 40 weeks CA, 6 seconds (Hahn et al., 1989). In general, the longest interval within an individual record is measured, rather than assessing an average of intervals. Although a prolongation of the interburst interval may be secondary to a CNS insult, it may also be due to the use of sedative medications such as morphine (Young and da Silva, 2000) and sufentanil (Nguyen et al., 2003).

### Episodes of Generalized and Regional Voltage Attenuation in Term Infants

Another finding of diffuse dysfunction in the term infant is the presence of generalized or regional episodes of voltage attenuation (**Fig. 6–4**). Although abnormal, this finding suggests relatively mild diffuse dysfunction compared with other findings listed later.

### Depression and Lack of Differentiation

Depressed beta activity, either focal or diffuse, is often the first manifestation of abnormal cortical function. After hypoxia–ischemia, faster frequencies tend to be depressed or obliterated. Lack of differentiation (i.e., the "undifferentiated EEG") refers to virtual or complete disappearance of the polyfrequency activity normally present (**Fig. 6–5**). A depressed and undifferentiated EEG background often accompanies other abnormalities (**Fig. 6–6**). However, in some instances, developmental milestones may persist (**Fig. 6–7**). A depressed and undifferentiated EEG in the newborn indicates that a severe brain insult has occurred. Disorders causing such an EEG include profound hypoxia–ischemia, severe metabolic disorders, infectious processes such as meningitis or encephalitis, cerebral hemorrhage, and intraventricular hemorrhage (IVH). A depressed and undifferentiated EEG within the first 24 hours after birth that persists signifies a poor prognosis.

### Suppression-Burst Pattern

The suppression-burst pattern represents an intermediate degree of diffuse brain disturbance between the depressed and undifferentiated EEG and electrocerebral silence. Activity during the bursts consists primarily of delta and theta frequencies, which at times is intermixed with sharp waves. The bursts are separated by periods of marked generalized voltage attenuation or electrocerebral silence (**Figs. 6–8 to 6–13**). Suppression-burst patterns persist unremittingly; no change in the EEG activity is seen during the entire recording, and the pattern does not react to painful stimuli. Some infants with the suppression-burst pattern may experience periodic slow myoclonic jerks (**Figs. 6–14 and 6–15**).

### Electrocerebral Silence

Electrocerebral silence represents the ultimate degree of depression and lack of differentiation in the neonate. The transition from a severely depressed and undifferentiated background to isoelectric may be difficult to determine (**Fig. 6–16**), and serial EEGs may be required to demonstrate a persistent degree of cortical inactivity (**Fig. 6–17**). An isoelectric EEG (i.e., "electrocerebral silence") is evidence of death only of the cortex, not of the brainstem, which, in the infant, may sustain vital functions for prolonged periods. Indeed, prolonged survival may occur in infants whose EEGs continue to show electrocerebral silence (Mizrahi et al., 1985).

### Specialized Generalized Patterns

#### Hypsarrhythmia

The classic hypsarrhythmic pattern as described by Gibbs and Gibbs (1952) rarely appears before 44 weeks CA. However, one modification of this pattern in the neonatal period is the suppression-burst variant (Hrachvoy et al., 1984), characterized by periodic bursts of high-voltage activity (**Fig. 6–15**). The bursts consist of asynchronous, high-voltage, slow activity mixed with multifocal spikes and sharp waves. The primary features that distinguish this variant of hypsarrhythmia are the periodicity of the bursts and the high voltage of the activity within the bursts.

Patients with infantile spasms and this variant of hypsarrhythmia have a poor prognosis for long-term outcome, regardless of whether the pattern develops in the neonatal period or in later months of life (Maheshwari and Jeavons, 1975). In addition, when this pattern does appear in the neonatal period, it is closely associated with the presence of inborn errors of metabolism, most notably nonketotic hyperglycinemia.

#### Holoprosencephaly

The term holoprosencephaly is applied to a spectrum of related cerebral malformations resulting from faulty diverticulation of the prosencephalon. The malformation varies in severity, from arhinencephaly (in which the olfactory bulbs and tracts are absent but the brain is otherwise normal) to alobar holoprosencephaly (in which lobes are not demarcated and the cerebrum is monoventricular, with or without a dorsal cyst). A variety of median facial defects (including cyclopia, orbital hypotelorism, cleft lip, cleft palate, and hypoplasia of the premaxilla) are associated with the cerebral malformations (DeMyer and Zeman, 1963; Yakovlev, 1959).

The EEG findings associated with holoprosencephaly were described by DeMyer and White (1964). They include (a) multifocal spike and polyspike activity mixed with slow waves; (b) periods of monorhythmic beta-, alpha-, theta-, or delta-frequency activity, occurring singly or in various combinations; (c) asynchrony between hemispheres; (d) isoelectric or relatively low voltage activity; (e) periodic patterns; and (f) lack of any normal organization (**Figs. 6–18 and 6–19**). These findings occur in various combinations in a single patient. Equally dramatic are the repeated and abrupt changes from one pattern to another, such that in a few minutes, most or all of the aforementioned features can be visualized. This constellation of findings is not seen in other disorders of infancy and is therefore diagnostic for holoprosencephaly. Infants with holoprosencephaly often have unusual or stereotyped movements suggestive of seizures. However, no correlation exists between these movements and EEG changes. The prognosis is poor; about 50% of infants die within the first month of life; about 80% will be dead within the first year.

## PATTERNS THAT MAY BE FOCAL OR GENERALIZED

### Sustained Rhythmic Alpha–Theta Activity

Sustained, rhythmic, 4- to 7-Hz activity (theta) and/or 8- to 10-Hz (alpha), 40- to 100-µV activity that is generalized or focal is an abnormal finding. However, precise correlations to specific etiologic factors have not, for the most part, been determined. This activity may occur almost continuously or paroxysmally in brief runs and may occur as only theta, alpha, or mixed activity (**Figs. 6–20 to 6–25**).

When alpha activity occurs focally, it is most prevalent in the central or temporal regions, where it may occur independently on the two sides. Although this activity may be most prominent in the awake state, it is usually present in all states and is accompanied by other abnormalities, such as abnormal sharp waves. Generalized rhythmic alpha and/or theta activity has been associated with various underlying abnormalities, most commonly congenital heart disease; however, it also may be seen in infants who have received CNS-active drugs such as diazepam and phenobarbital (Hrachovy and O'Donnell, 1996). It is important to distinguish this pattern from the alpha seizure pattern (see Chapter 7).

### Sustained Rhythmic Delta Activity

In some instances, bifrontal slow (delta) activity is considered an abnormal finding. Abnormal bifrontal slow activity can be differentiated from normal bifrontal slow activity by its presence in all stages of sleep and wakefulness and its unrelenting character (**Fig. 6–26**). Abnormal rhythmic slow (delta) activity also may be present in the occipital regions bilaterally (**Fig. 6–27**).

## FOCAL ABNORMALITIES

### Periodic Complexes
Focal periodic and quasiperiodic discharges in a newborn's EEG have been reported to be suggestive of neonatal herpes simplex encephalitis (HSVE) (Mizrahi and Tharp, 1982) (**Fig. 6–28**). Although such periodic discharges may be associated with HSVE, such discharges also may be interpreted as electrical seizures of the depressed-brain type (see Chapter 7). In addition, periodic discharges are not, however, peculiar to HSVE and may occur with various other CNS insults such as infarction (Scher and Beggarly, 1989).

### Unilateral Depression of Background Activity
Mild shifting asymmetry of the background EEG activity between hemispheres is a common finding in the newborn, particularly during quiet sleep. However, an abnormal finding is a marked voltage asymmetry of background rhythms between hemispheres that persists in all states (**Figs. 6–13 and 6–29 to 6–31**). Unilateral depression may occur in association with a wide range of structural cerebral lesions such as infarction, hemorrhage, focal cystic lesions, and rarely, congenital malformation. In addition, other intracranial abnormalities such as subdural fluid collections may be associated with this EEG finding. However, focal depression of the background activity may persist for variable periods after electrical seizures. A marked asymmetry of the background activity also may result from nonintracranial causes such as subgaleal swelling, scalp edema, or technical error.

### Focal Slow Activity
Just as in older infants, the finding of focal slow activity that persists at a specific site may indicate the presence of a focal destructive lesion such as infarction, hemorrhage, or, more specific to neonates, congenital anomalies of the brain (**Fig. 6–32**).

### Central Positive Sharp Waves
These waves are 50- to 250-μV surface-positive transients lasting 100 to 250 milliseconds and occurring either unilaterally or bilaterally in the central regions (**Figs. 6–33 to 6–37**). A lower-voltage aftergoing surface-negative component

may be present. The waves usually occur singly or in brief runs. Central positive sharp waves are not epileptiform discharges, and the physiological processes causing them remain unknown. They have been described most notably in infants with IVH (Blume and Dreyfus-Brisac, 1982; Cukier et al., 1972; Lomboso, 1982; Tharp et al., 1981) and white-matter necrosis (periventricular leukomalacia) (Lomboso, 1982; Marret et al., 1986; Novotny et al., 1987); as well as other conditions, including meningitis, hydrocephalus, aminoaciduria (Tharp, 1980), and asphyxia (da Costa and Lombroso, 1980). Current thought is that central positive sharp waves are specific not for IVH but rather for white-matter necrosis, which may result from a variety of insults, including IVH (Novotny et al., 1987). In addition, the abundance and rate of recurrence of central positive sharp waves within a single record of an infant appears to correlate with long-term neurologic outcome; a rate of greater than two per second has been reported to be associated with a poor outcome (Blume and Dreyfus-Brisac, 1982).

### Temporal Sharp Waves
The problems of determining whether focal temporal sharp waves are normal or abnormal have been previously discussed (see Chapter 5). Whereas some sharp waves occurring in the temporal regions are considered normal, others may not meet the criteria to be called abnormal and are thus of questionable significance. However, some temporal sharp waves are clearly abnormal. Criteria for abnormality include morphology, polarity, rate of recurrence, and persistence at one site (**Figs. 6–38 and 6–39**).

### Extratemporal Focal Sharp Waves
Abnormal sharp waves that appear as slow sharp transients or rapid spikes may occur in the frontal (**Figs. 6–40 to 6–46**), central (**Figs. 6–47 to 6–49**), and occipital (**Figs. 6–50 to 6–52**) regions. When persistently focal, they may indicate focal brain injury, although often no well-defined structural lesion can be documented by neuroimaging.

### Multifocal Sharp Waves
As already noted, sharp waves in the newborn EEG are common, with certain sharp-wave activity being considered normal. Multiple foci of high-voltage,

long-duration, sharp-wave activity are commonly seen in infants who have had a diffuse CNS insult (**Figs. 6–53 to 6–56**). Such abnormal sharp waves usually predominate in the temporal regions and may persist over one hemisphere. Multifocal sharp waves usually accompany various other EEG abnormalities, including depressed and undifferentiated background activity and episodes of attenuation. However, multifocal sharp waves may be the only abnormality after a CNS insult and also may be the last remaining evidence of CNS dysfunction in serial tracings. This abnormality is usually maximal in quiet sleep, and in some infants, it may occur only in this state (**Fig. 6–2**). Multifocal sharp waves cannot be used as evidence that a seizure has occurred or will occur, because the sharp waves do not show a significant association with neonates with seizures.

## LIST OF FIGURES

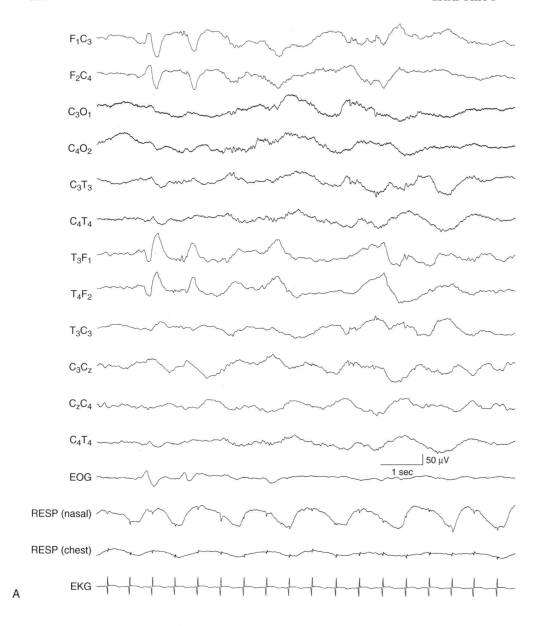

**FIG. 6–1. Internal dyschronism. A:** The developmental features of the EEG in this term infant in transitional sleep are consistent with a CA of 38 to 40 weeks and are within the range of normal variation.

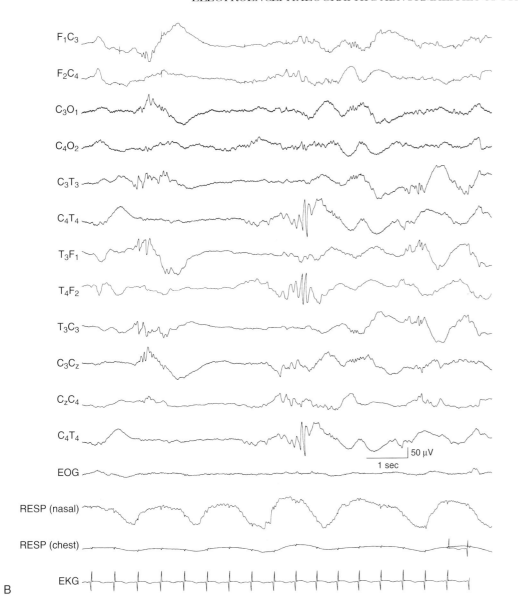

**FIG. 6–1.** *(Continued)* **B:** In deep non–rapid eye movement (NREM) sleep, during the same recording of the infant, the developmental features of the EEG are consistent with the CA of 33 weeks, with central beta–delta complexes, temporal alpha bursts, and a discontinuous background. This NREM sleep recording also is without abnormalities.

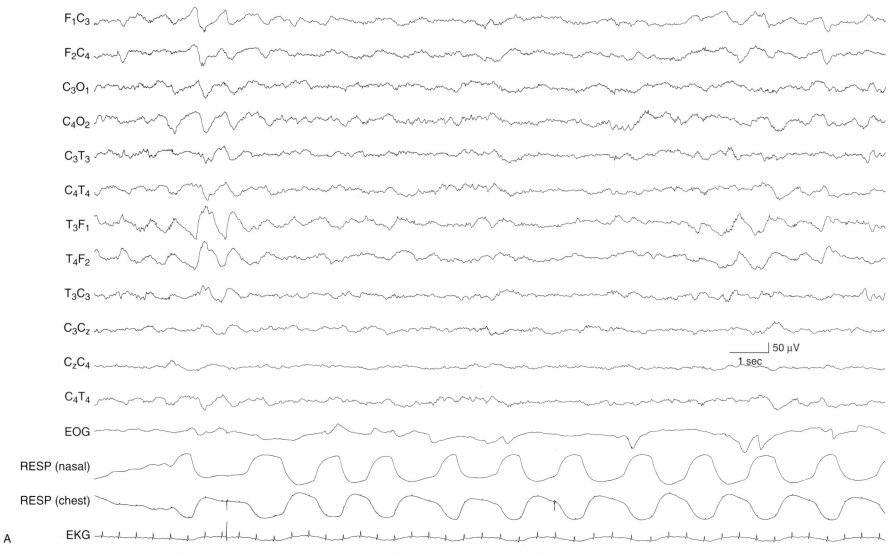

**FIG. 6–2. State-dependent abnormality of the EEG. A:** The awake EEG of this term infant, suspected of having hypoxic-ischemic encephalopathy, is within the range of normal variation, and its developmental features are consistent with that CA.

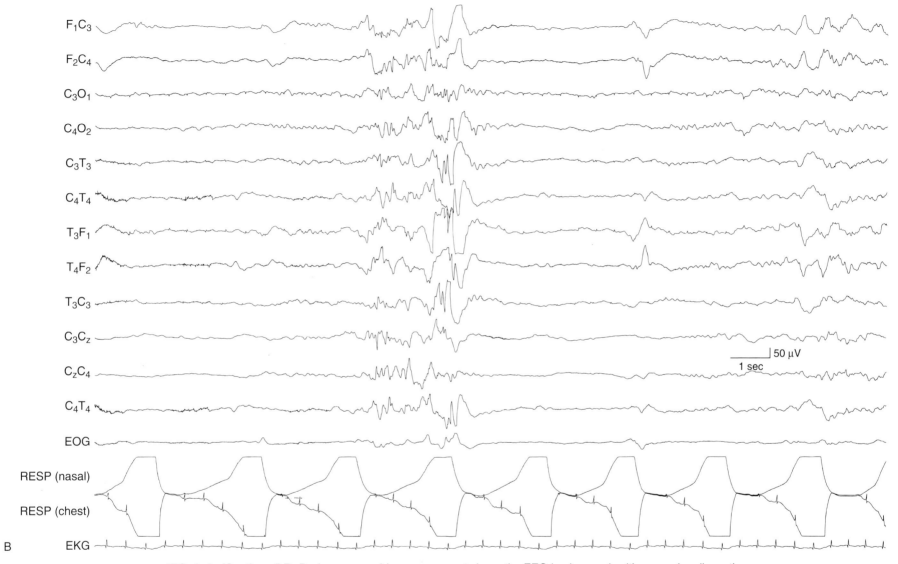

**FIG. 6–2.** *(Continued)* **B:** During non–rapid eye movement sleep, the EEG is abnormal, with excessive discontinuity, asynchronous activity including sharp waves and spikes, and no well-defined developmental milestones. This differs from internal dyschronism, because the features of the sleep recording are abnormal.

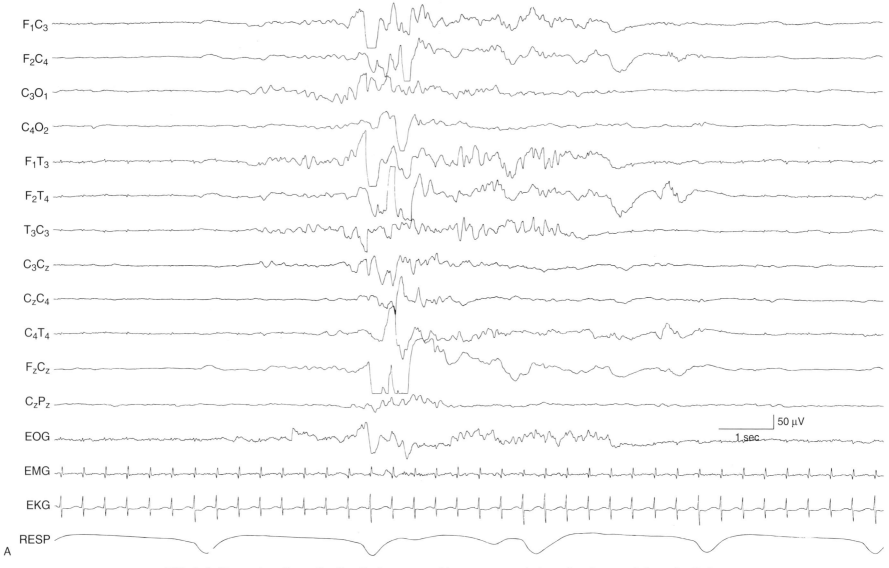

**FIG. 6–3. Excessive discontinuity.** During non–rapid eye movement sleep, the degree of discontinuity is excessive for the infant's CA of 35 weeks. This is shown in two contiguous segments **(A)** and **(B)**. In addition, there is an absence of beta–delta complexes. This infant was found to have grade III intraventicular hemorrhage bilaterally.

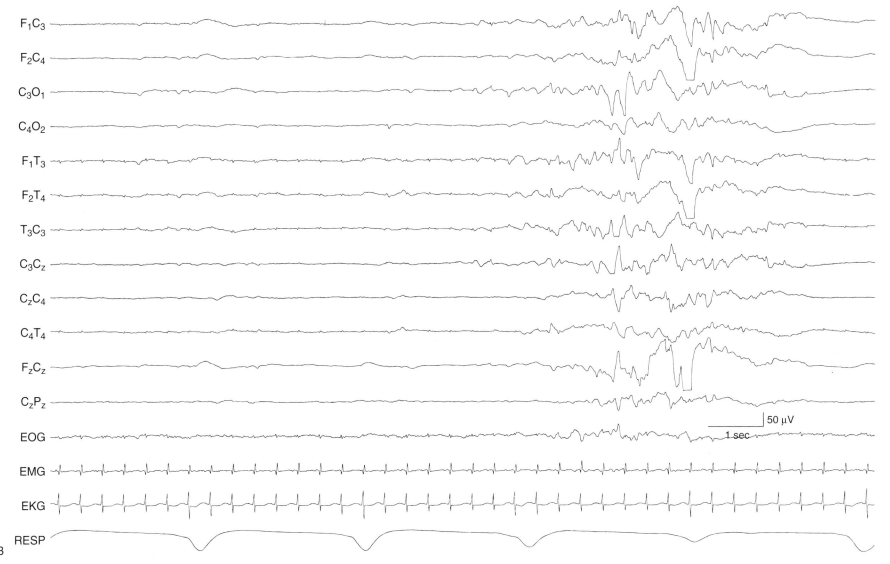

**FIG. 6–3.** *(Continued)*

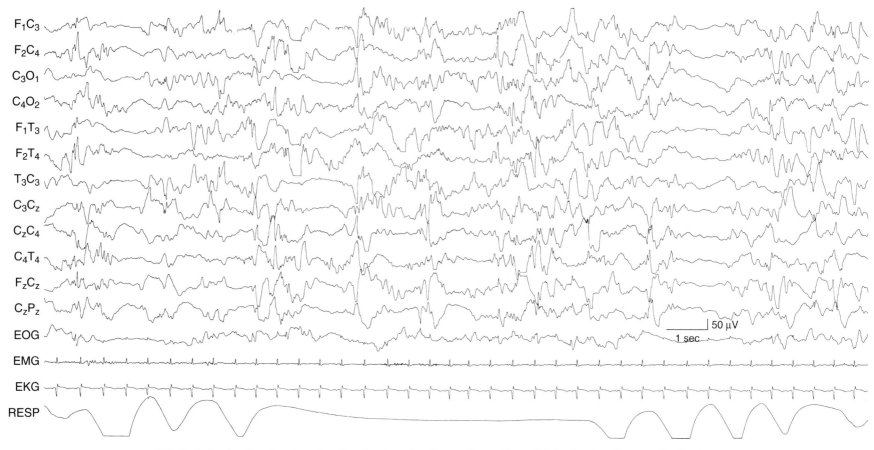

**FIG. 6–4. Generalized and regional episodes of voltage attenuation.** Brief episodes of generalized voltage attenuation lasting 1 to 2 seconds and episodes of similar character and duration appear independently in leads from the left and right hemispheres. The background activity also is abnormal with multifocal sharp waves. The EEG is from a 40-week CA infant who is lethargic and with computed tomography neuroimaging findings of bi-parietal white-matter lucencies. No specific etiology was identified.

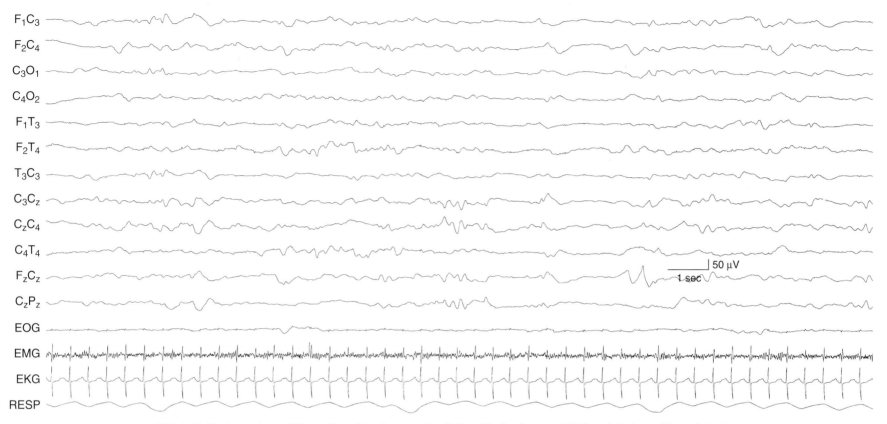

**FIG. 6–5. Moderately undifferentiated background activity.** The background EEG activity is undifferentiated, with a lack of developmental milestones, a lack of faster frequencies, and brief episodes of generalized voltage attenuation. The EEG comprises almost exclusively moderate-voltage slow activity. The infant is 43-week CA with the inborn error of metabolism, methylmalonic acidemia.

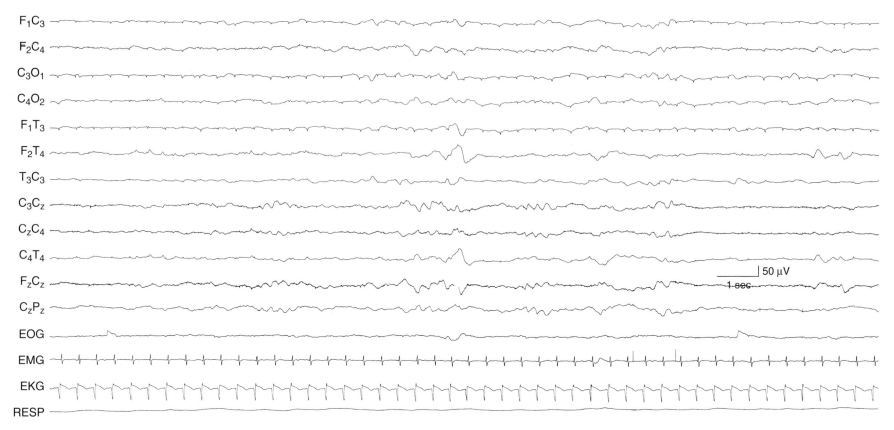

**FIG. 6–6. Undifferentiated background activity with periods of generalized voltage attenuation.** The background activity is low in voltage with no alpha or beta activity. Periods of generalized voltage attenuation appear early and late in the sample. The EEG is from a 41-week CA infant with renal failure and metabolic acidosis. The patient was on renal dialysis at the time of recording.

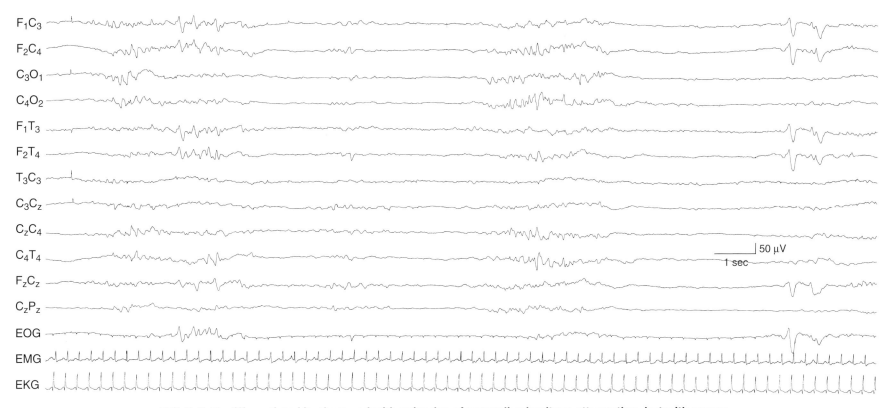

**FIG. 6–7. Undifferentiated background with episodes of generalized voltage attenuation, but with preservation of some developmental milestones.** The background activity is depressed and undifferentiated with intermittent rhythmic theta activity between episodes of generalized voltage attenuation. Early in the sample, abnormal sharp waves occur in the frontal regions. However, later in the sample, normal frontal sharp transients are present. Such findings can be distinguished from a suppression-burst pattern when other portions of the EEG are continuous and by the presence of normal developmental milestones. The EEG is from a 39-week CA infant with congenital heart disease and chronic hypoxemia.

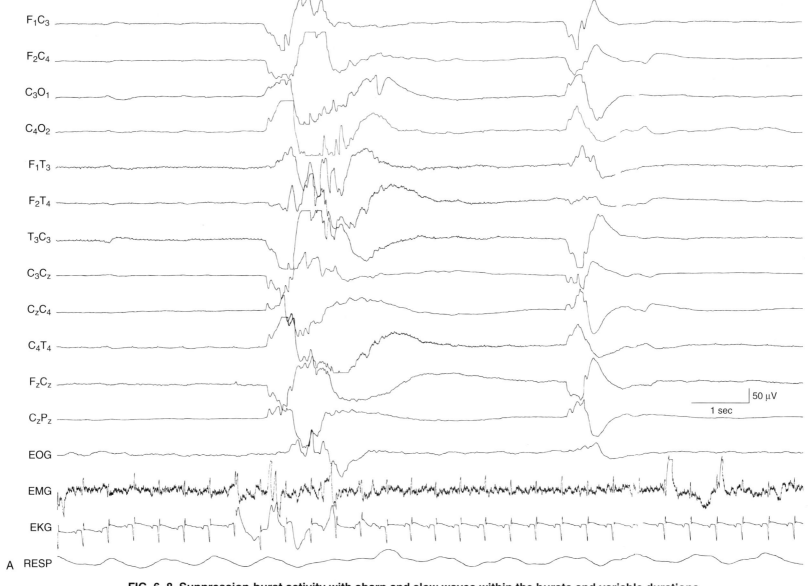

**FIG. 6–8. Suppression-burst activity with sharp and slow waves within the bursts and variable durations between bursts.** The brief bursts are characterized by high-voltage slow activity with superimposed theta and alpha activity. The bursts are followed by high-voltage very slow wave transients. The periods of suppression are variable in these contiguous samples **(A, B)**, lasting from 3 seconds to >10 seconds. This EEG was recorded from a 35-week CA infant who was lethargic with hypoxic-ischemic encephalopathy, microcephaly, and the finding of periventricular leukomalacia on head computed tomography.

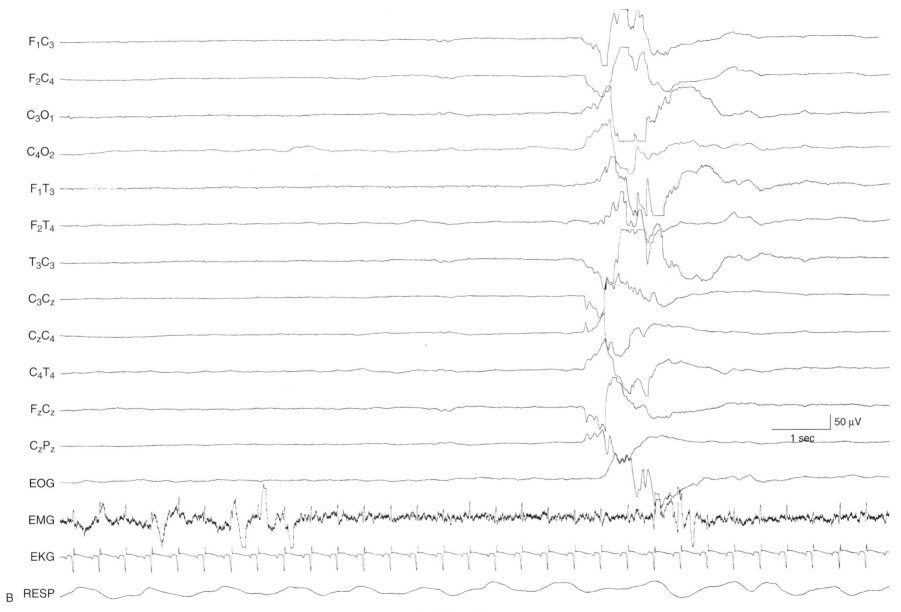

**FIG. 6–8.** *(Continued)*

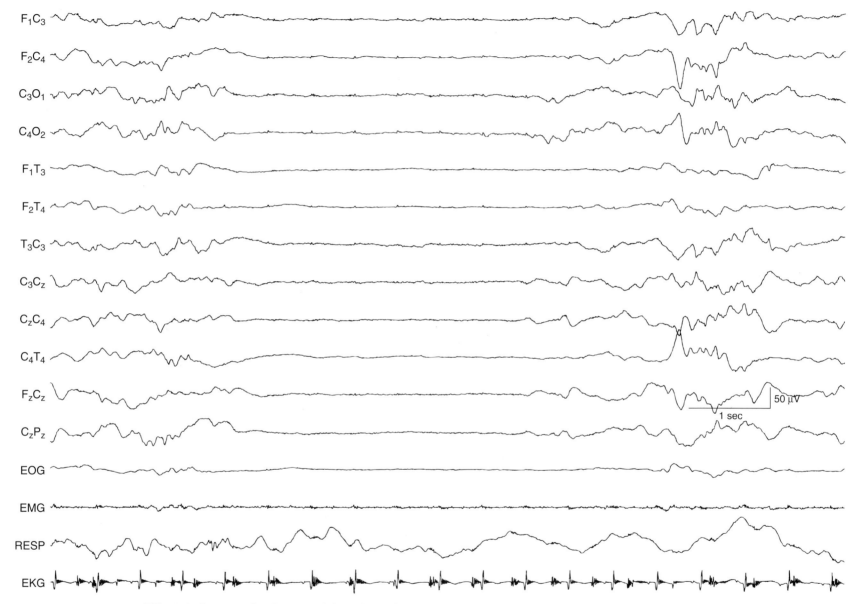

**FIG. 6–9. Suppression-burst activity with activity of normal character within the bursts.** The bursts are characterized by moderate-voltage activity of mixed slow and faster frequencies, which, if continuous, would be considered normal for this term infant. However, the background activity is suppression-burst. This term infant had meconium aspiration, required ventilatory support and, by the time of this recording, was maintained with extracorporeal membrane oxygenation.

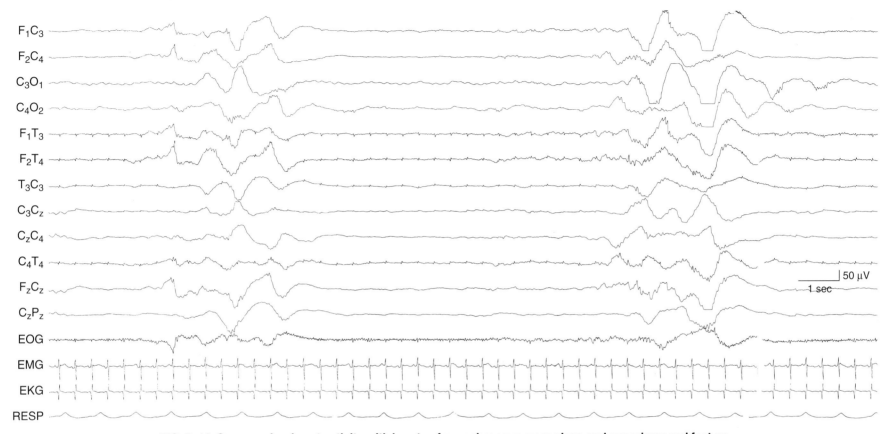

**FIG. 6–10. Suppression-burst activity with bursts of asynchronous, very slow, and superimposed fast activity.** The bursts are characterized by high-voltage, very slow activity with superimposed very low voltage faster activity. This occurs asynchronously on the two sides. The infant is 37 weeks CA, with hypoxic-ischemic encephalopathy, multisystem organ failure, and intracerebral hemorrhage on the left—in this instance with no consistent lateralizing findings on EEG.

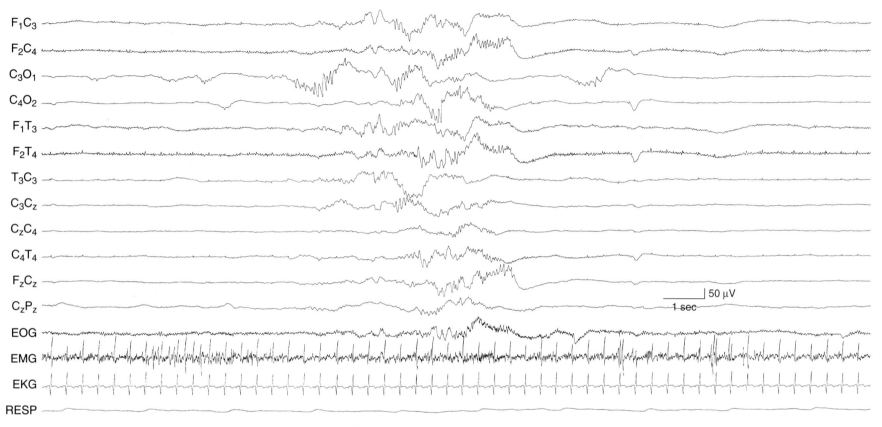

**FIG. 6–11. Suppression-burst activity with predominance of fast activity within the bursts.** Runs of moderate-voltage fast activity are present asynchronously on the two sides during periods of bursting. The infant is 35 weeks CA with metabolic acidosis, cardiac failure, pulmonary edema, peritonitis, and microcephaly.

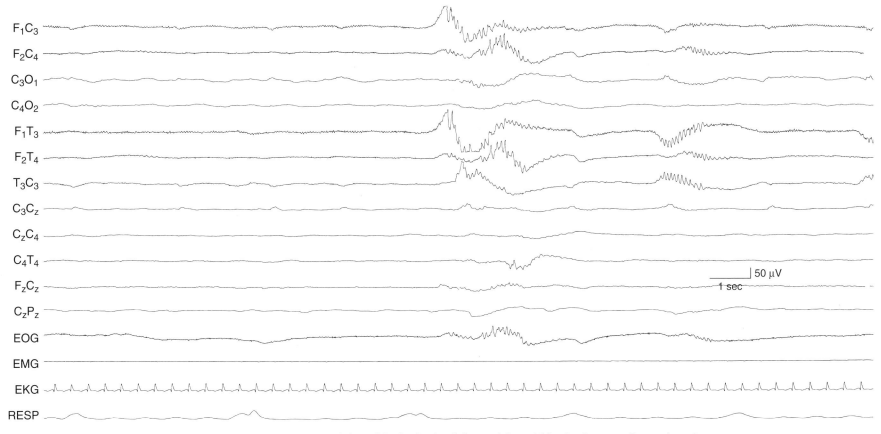

**FIG. 6–12. Suppression-burst activity with rhythmic alpha activity within the bursts.** Runs of moderate-voltage rhythmic alpha activity in the frontotemporal regions appear asynchronously within the bursts of this suppression-burst recording. This EEG is from a 35-week CA infant with hypoxic-ischemic encephalopathy.

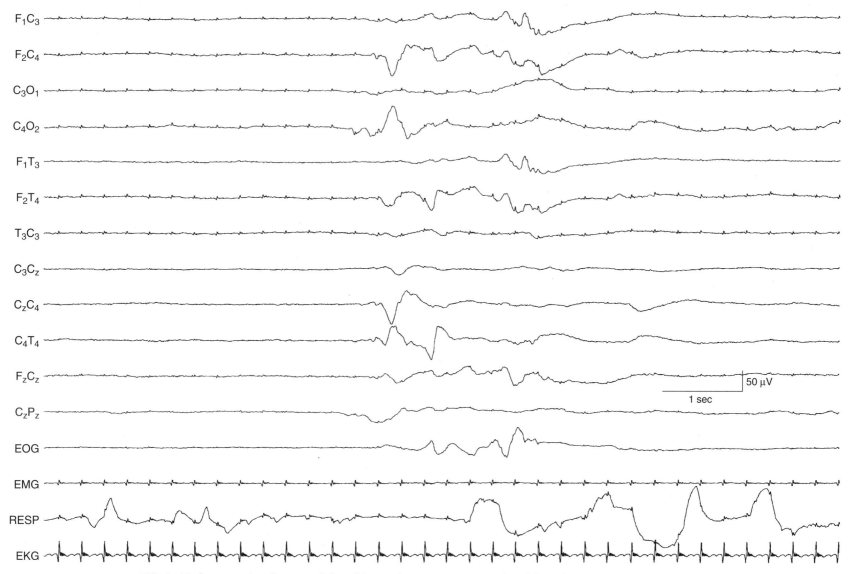

**FIG. 6–13. Suppression-burst activity with persistent asymmetry of activity within the bursts.** The bursts are characterized by moderate-voltage theta and delta activity. Persistent voltage asymmetry of the bursts is present with the amplitudes of waves lower in leads from the left centrotemporal region compared with homologous regions on the right. This term infant was born by emergency cesarean section, had persistent cyanosis, and required support by extracorporeal membrane oxygenation. The asymmetry on EEG is most likely owing to dependent scalp edema on the left.

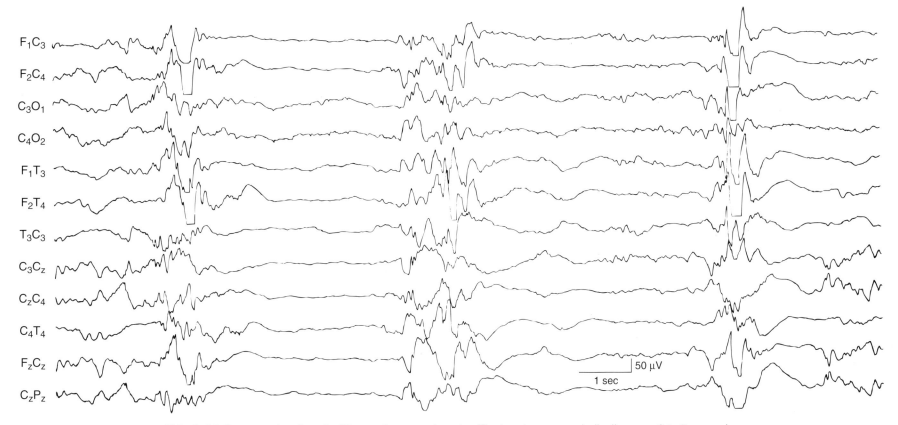

**FIG. 6–14. Suppression-burst with synchronous bursts.** The bursts recur periodically every 3 to 5 seconds, but are brief, lasting 1 to 2 seconds, with fairly synchronous activity on the two sides. This term infant experienced generalized myoclonic and focal clonic seizures with the eventual finding of the inborn error of metabolism, non-ketotic hyperglycinemia. (From Mizrahi EM, Kellaway P. *Diagnosis and management of neonatal seizures.* Philadelphia: Lippincott-Raven, 1998:181, with permission.)

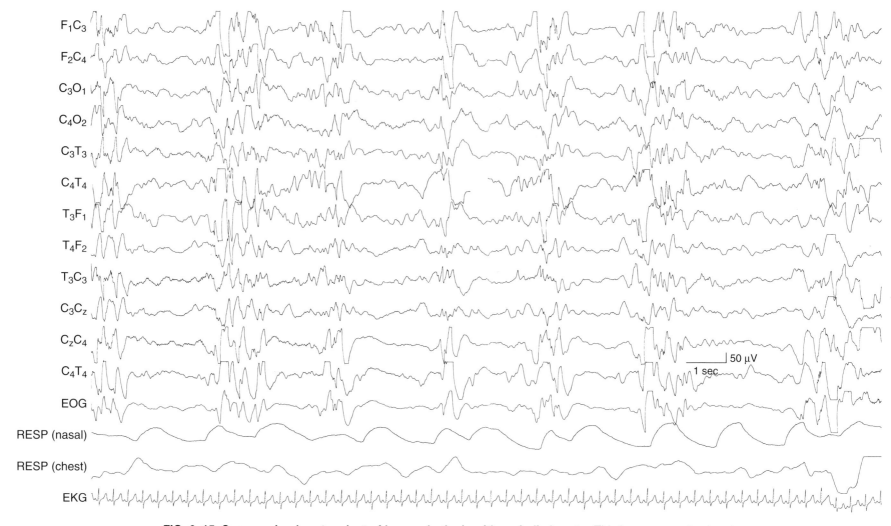

**FIG. 6–15. Suppression-burst variant of hypsarrhythmia with periodic bursts.** This is a suppression-burst variant of hypsarrhythmia in a 43-week CA infant with an inborn error of metabolism and a clinical diagnosis of early myoclonic encephalopathy. The infant had infantile spasms accompanied by generalized voltage attenuations in the EEG (not shown).

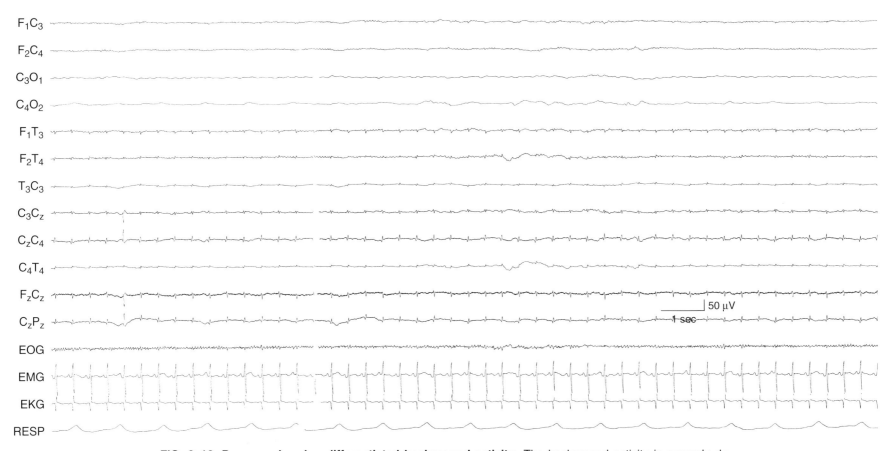

**FIG. 6–16. Depressed and undifferentiated background activity.** The background activity is severely depressed and undifferentiated in all regions with only electrocardiogram artifact and occasional very low voltage slow waves present. This EEG is from a 37-week CA infant with hypoxic–ischemic encephalopathy (Apgar scores, 1 at 1 minute, 1 at 5 minutes), multiorgan system failure, and intracerebral hemorrhage.

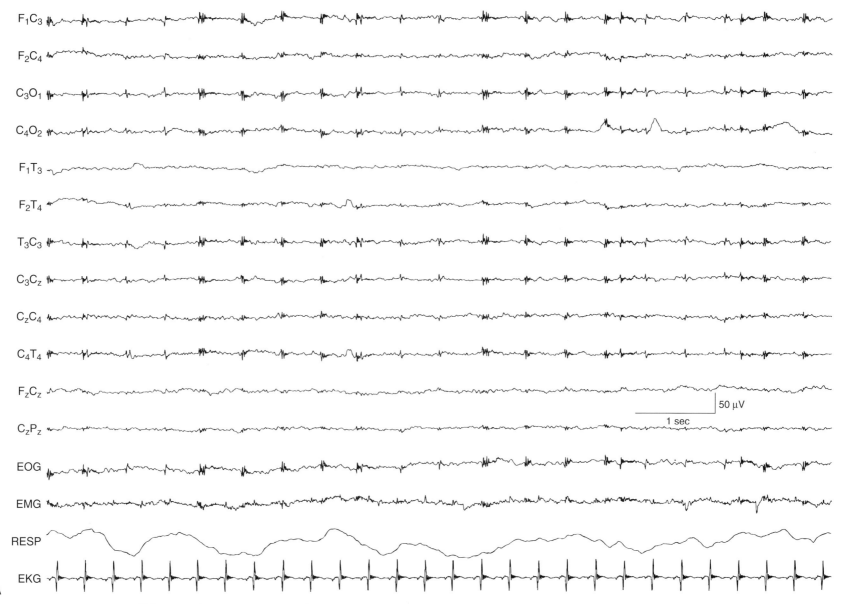

**FIG. 6–17. Depressed and undifferentiated background activity evolving to suppression-burst activity. A:**
The EEG is depressed and undifferentiated with artifact from electrocardiogram and extracorporeal membrane oxygenation instrumentation. This EEG was recorded on day 3 of life from this term infant with hypoxic-ischemic encephalopathy.

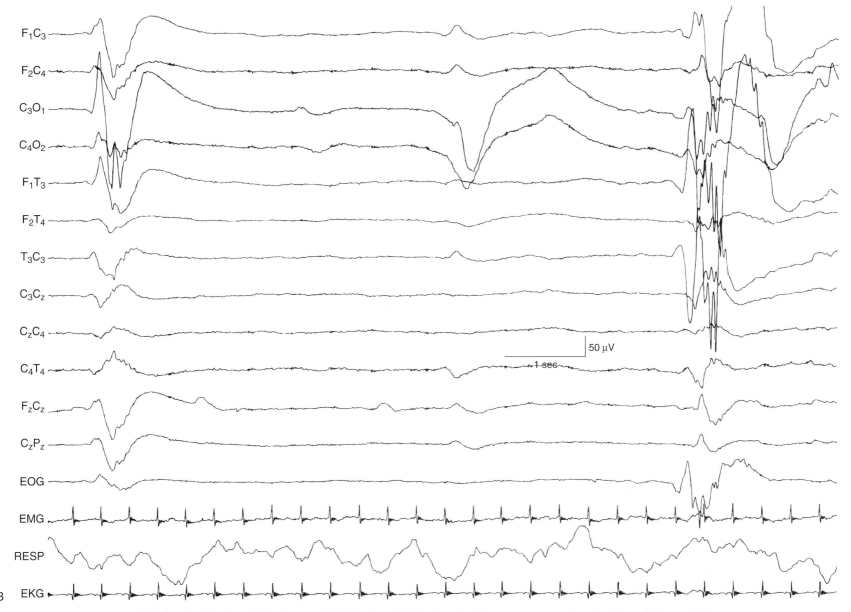

**FIG. 6–17.** *(Continued)* **B:** On day 10 of life, the EEG had evolved to a suppression-burst pattern. Although this represented a change in the EEG findings with some improvement, the rate of improvement and the change to only suppression-burst suggested a poor prognosis in terms of neurologic outcome.

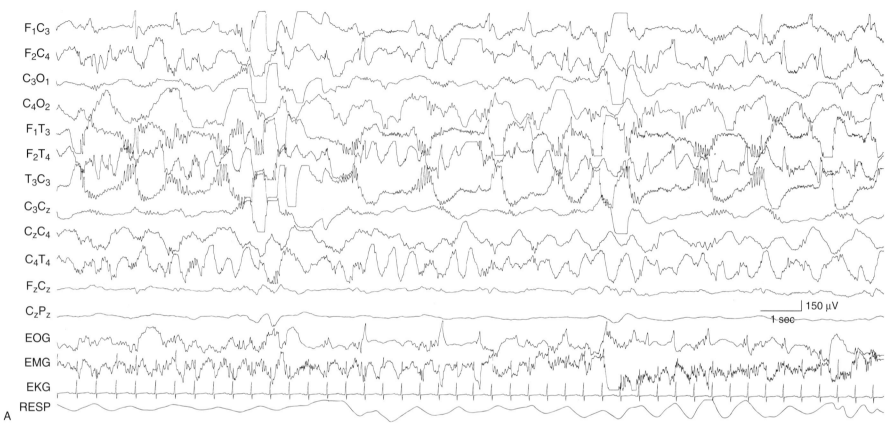

**FIG. 6–18. Dynamic pattern of holoprosencephaly.** These are samples from a single EEG recorded from a term infant with holoprosencephaly diagnosed by clinical and magnetic resonance imaging findings. **A:** Multiple foci of spike and polyspike activity are mixed with slow-wave activity, with independent delta activity with superimposed beta activity.

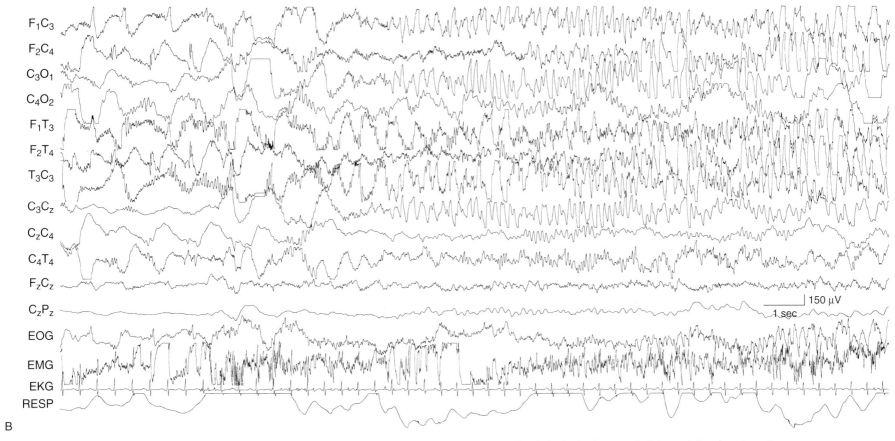

**FIG. 6–18.** *(Continued)* **B:** A sudden transition occurs to sustained rhythmic theta and alpha activity. *(continued)*

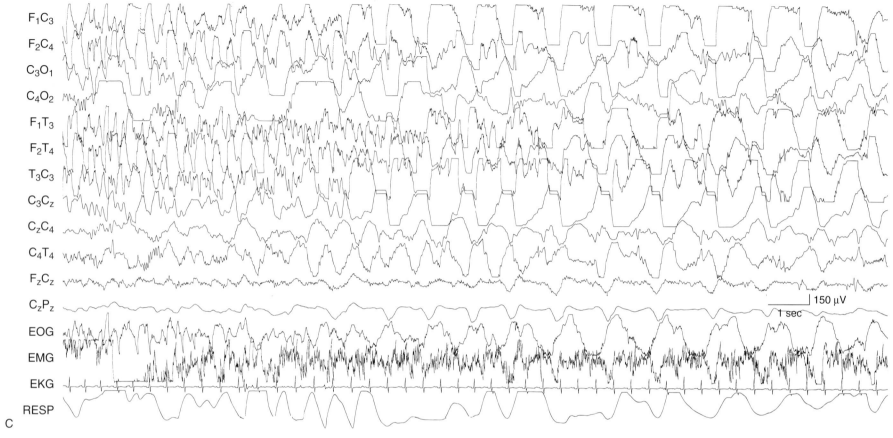

**FIG. 6–18.** *(Continued)* **C:** A sudden transition to high-voltage rhythmic slow activity is seen predominantly on the left. Note the voltage calibration that indicates the very high voltage of this activity.

**FIGURES CONTINUE ON THE NEXT PAGE**

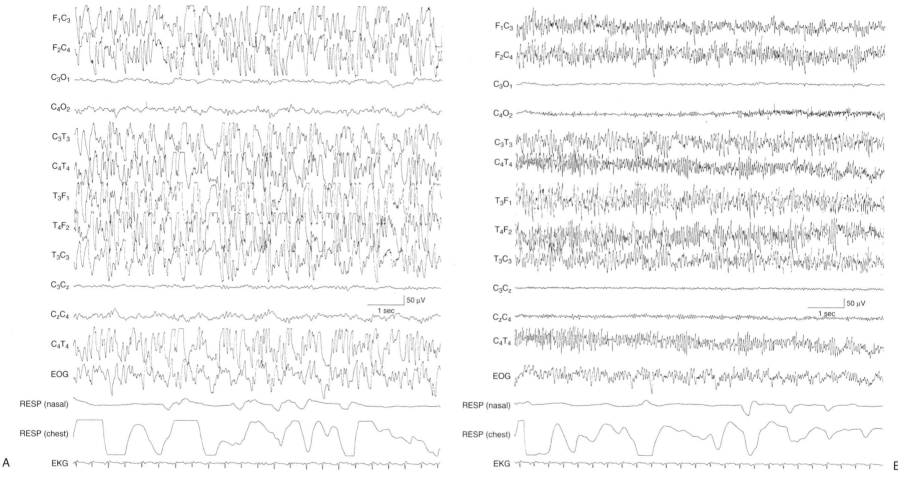

**FIG. 6–19. Dynamic pattern of holoprosencephaly with persistent focal features.** The EEG features that are typical in infants with holoprosencephaly are present in this term infant who, as part of the brain malformation, also has a dorsal cystic lesion that is characterized on EEG by marked depression of activity in the affected regions. **A:** High-voltage, rhythmic, alpha and theta frequency activity is mixed with some slower waveforms. **B:** High-voltage, rhythmic fast activity is present.

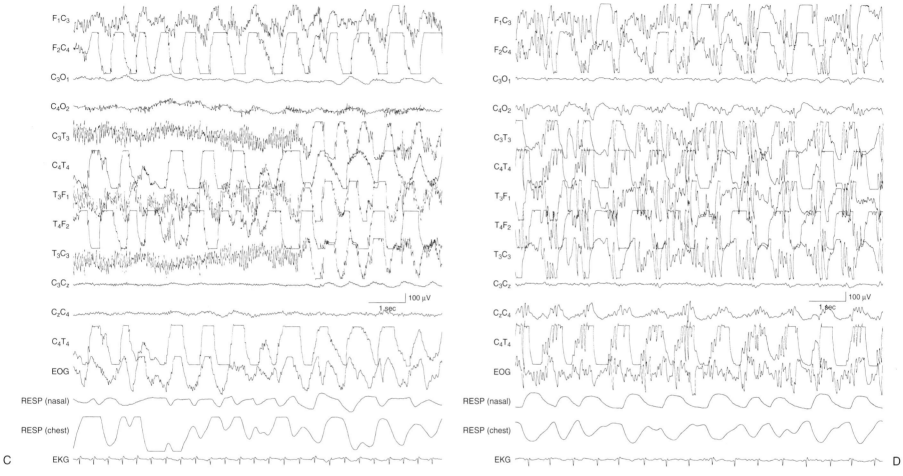

**FIG. 6–19.** *(Continued)* **C:** High-voltage very slow activity is present on the right with the persistence of fast activity on the left until a sudden transition to slower frequencies on that side. **D:** Asynchronous, high-voltage very slow activity with superimposed fast activity is present.

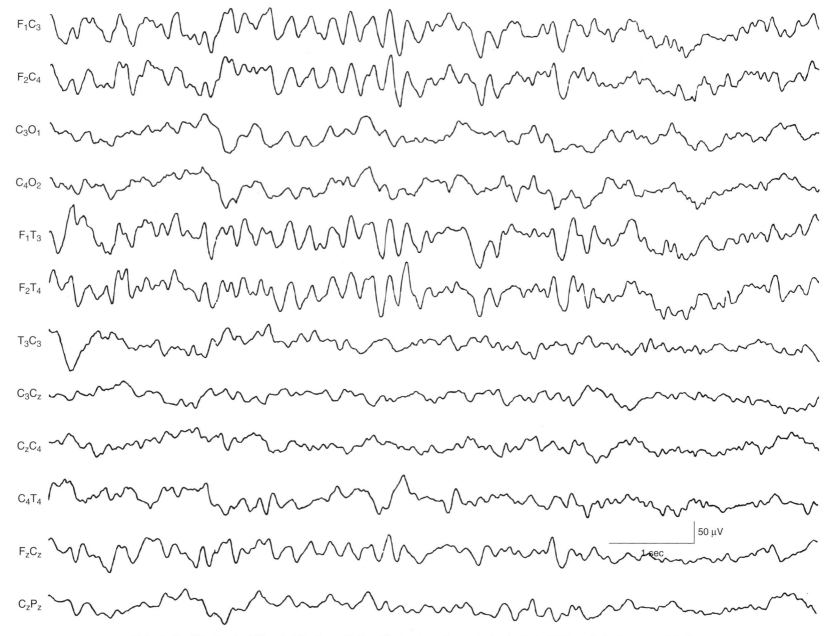

**FIG. 6–20. Rhythmic bifrontal theta activity.** Moderate-voltage rhythmic 5- to 6-Hz activity is present in the frontal regions bilaterally in the EEG that is otherwise normal in this term infant.

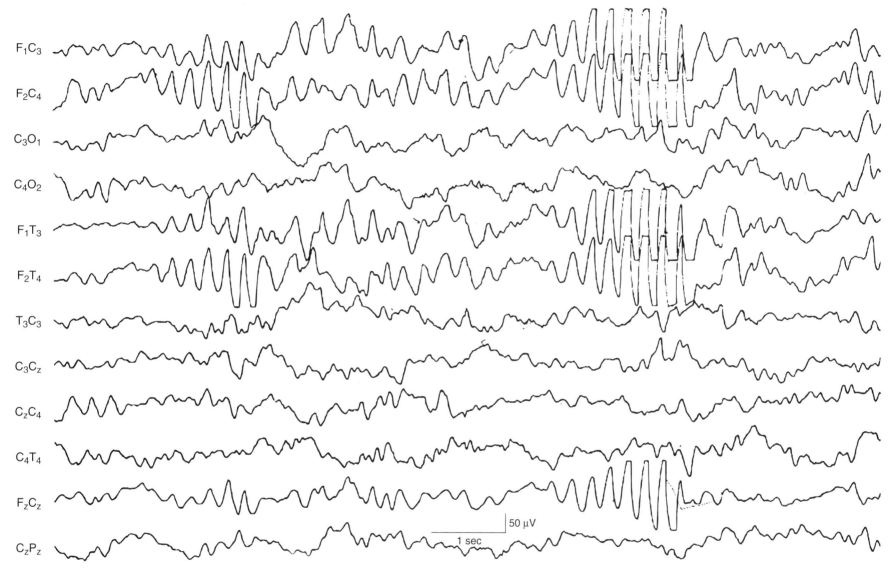

**FIG. 6–21. Paroxysmal bifrontal theta activity.** Paroxysmal moderately high voltage 5- to 6-Hz activity appears in the frontal regions bilaterally. The EEG is otherwise normal in this term infant.

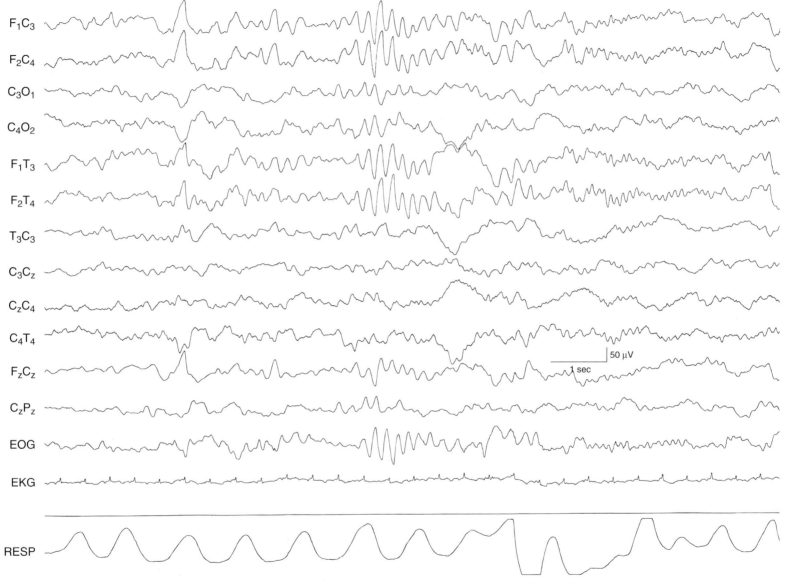

**FIG. 6–22. Rhythmic bifrontal theta activity followed by rhythmic bifrontal alpha activity.** There is a burst of rhythmic high voltage 5- to 6-Hz activity in the frontal regions bilaterally followed by a run of low-voltage rhythmic 8- to 9-Hz activity. The background EEG activity is otherwise normal in this term infant.

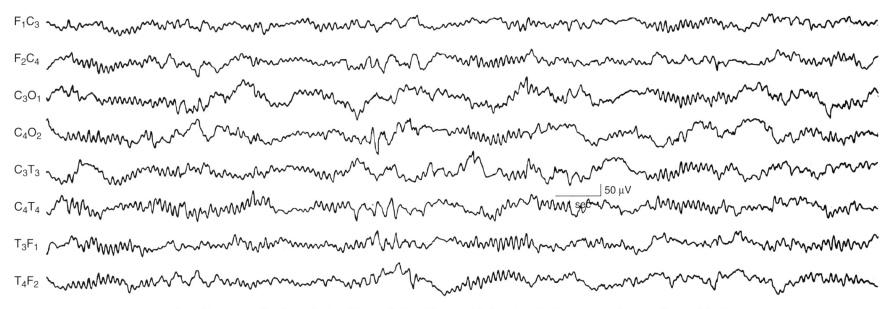

**FIG. 6–23. Generalized rhythmic alpha activity with variable interhemispheric asynchrony.** Runs of rhythmic 8- to 9-Hz activity occur both synchronously and asynchronously in the left and right central regions in a term infant with a chromosomal abnormality and multiple congenital anomalies. (From Hrachovy RA, Mizrahi EM, Kellaway P. Electroencephalography of the newborn. In: Daly DD, Pedley TA, eds. *Current practice of clinical electroencephalography,* 2nd ed. New York: Raven Press, 1990:201–241, with permission.)

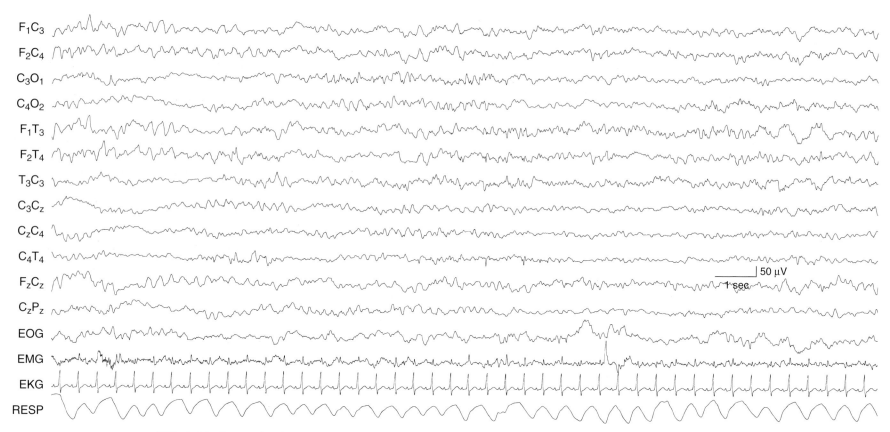

**FIG. 6–24. Generalized rhythmic alpha and theta activity.** Runs of 8- to 9-Hz activity are mixed with 5- to 6-Hz activity in all regions in the EEG of this term infant with congenital heart disease.

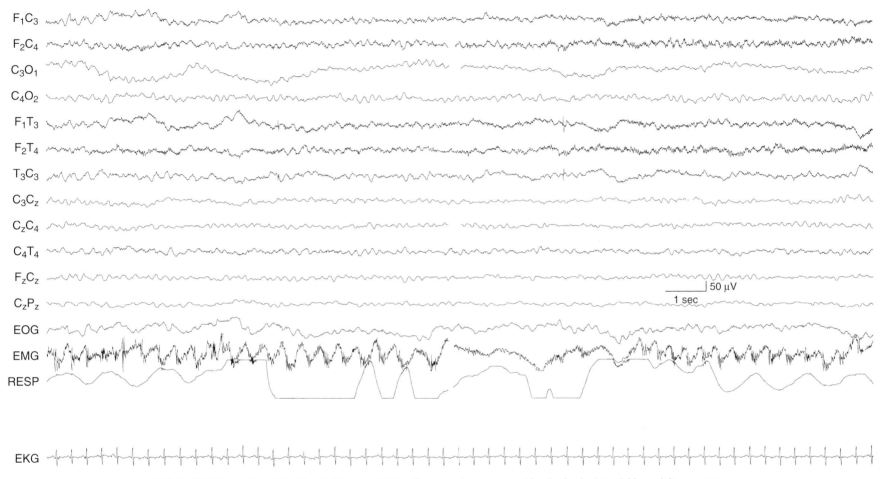

**FIG. 6–25. Generalized rhythmic theta activity.** Sustained, monomorphic, rhythmic 5- to 6-Hz activity appears chiefly in anterior regions in this term infant with the inborn error of metabolism, citrullinemia.

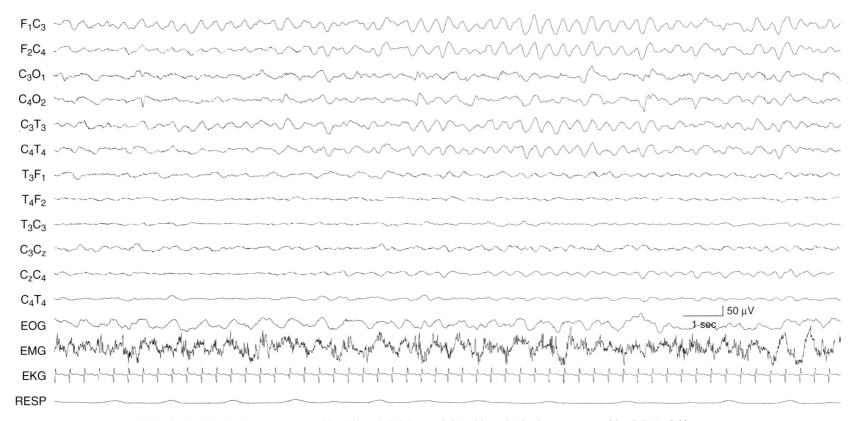

**FIG. 6–26. Rhythmic, monomorphic, bifrontal delta activity.** Monorhythmic, monomorphic, 2.5- to 3-Hz activity in the frontal regions bilaterally and the background activity is depressed in this term infant with nonaccidental head injury.

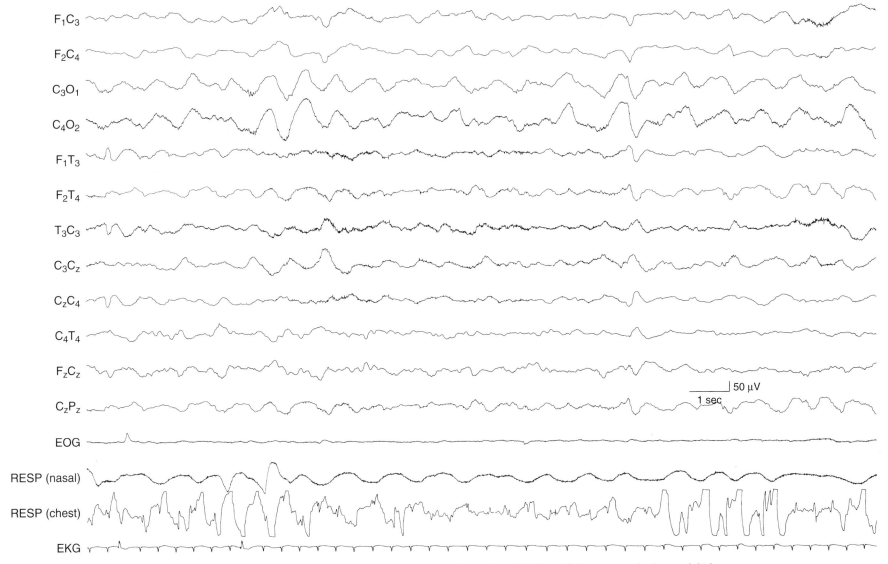

**FIG. 6–27. Rhythmic biooccipital slow activity.** High-voltage, 1- to 1.5-Hz activity appears in the occipital regions of the EEG of this term infant. The background activity is undifferentiated.

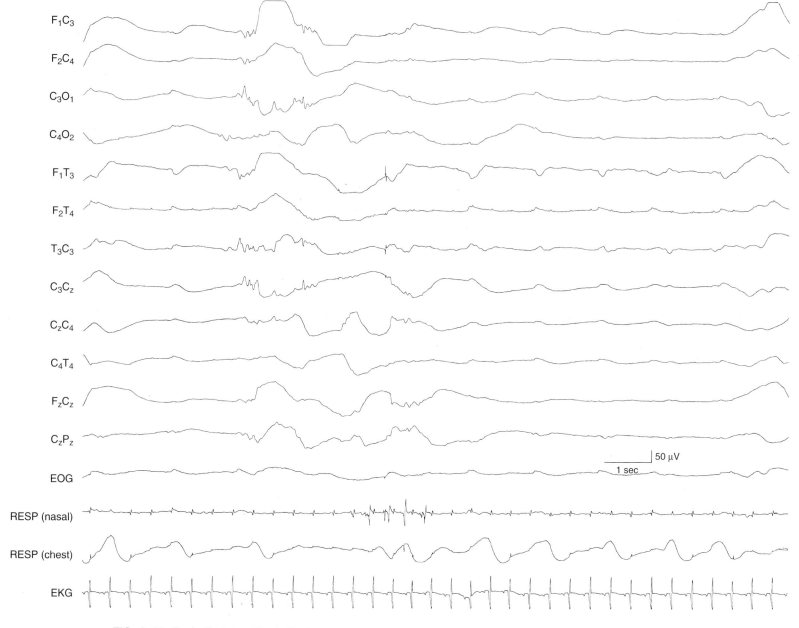

**FIG. 6–28. Periodic lateralized discharges associated with herpes simplex virus encephalitis.** Low-voltage, slow transients recur periodically in the left temporal region in this term infant with laboratory-confirmed herpes simplex virus encephalitis. The background activity is depressed and undifferentiated, with randomly occurring low voltage sharp waves in the left central region.

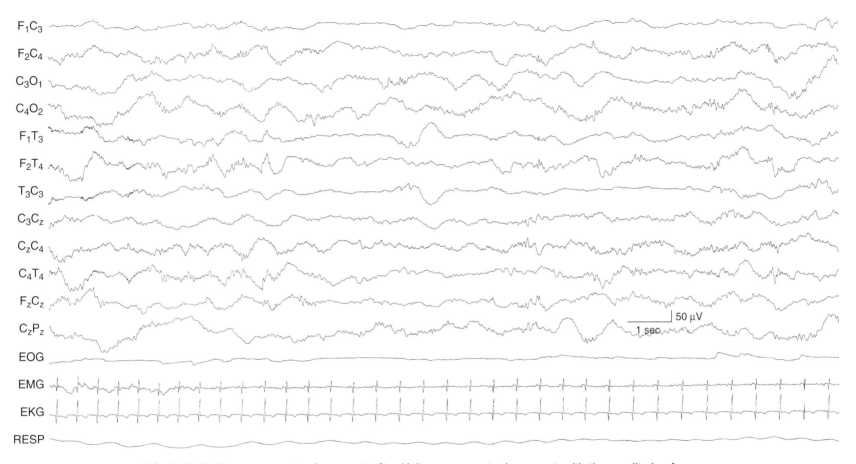

**FIG. 6–29. Voltage asymmetry in prematurity.** Voltage asymmetry is present, with the amplitude of waves lower in the leads from the left hemisphere compared with the right. The background activity on the right shows beta–delta complexes. This 35- to 36-week CA infant had a left frontoparietal intracerebral hemorrhage and an intraventricular hemorrhage with involvement of the germinal matrix on the left.

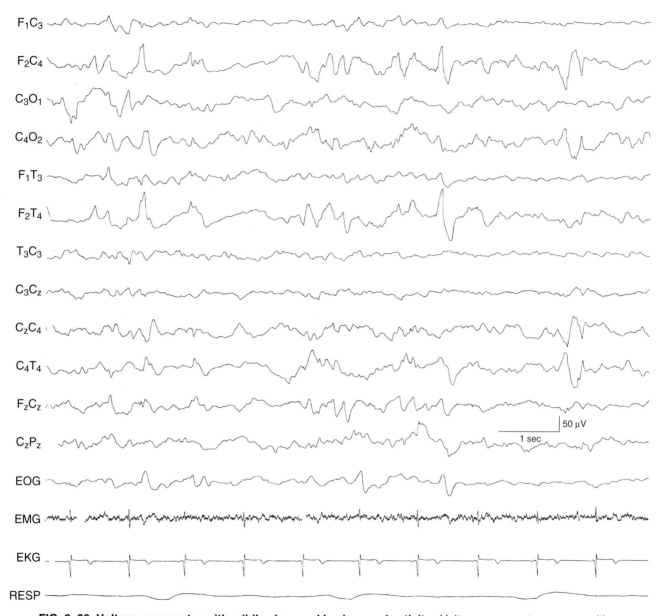

**FIG. 6–30. Voltage asymmetry with mildly abnormal background activity.** Voltage asymmetry appears with the amplitude of waves lower on the left compared with that in homologous regions on the right. Although frontal sharp transients (normal developmental milestones) persist on the right, the background activity is abnormal with a lack of faster frequencies. This term infant had a left frontoparietal intracerebral hemorrhage.

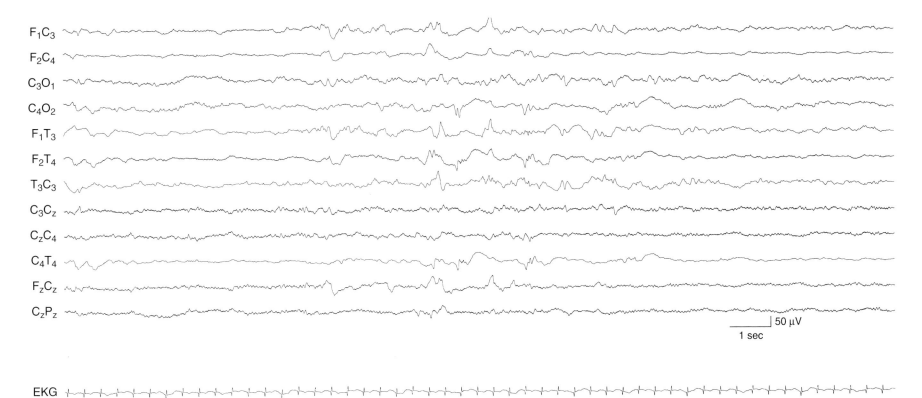

**FIG. 6–31. Voltage asymmetry associated with abnormal background activity.** A voltage asymmetry is seen with the amplitude of waves lower in leads from the right centrotemporal region compared with the homologous region on the left. Random moderate-voltage sharp waves are present bilaterally. The background activity is low in voltage. The infant is term with a right parietal infarction and diagnosis of hypoxic-ischemic encephalopathy.

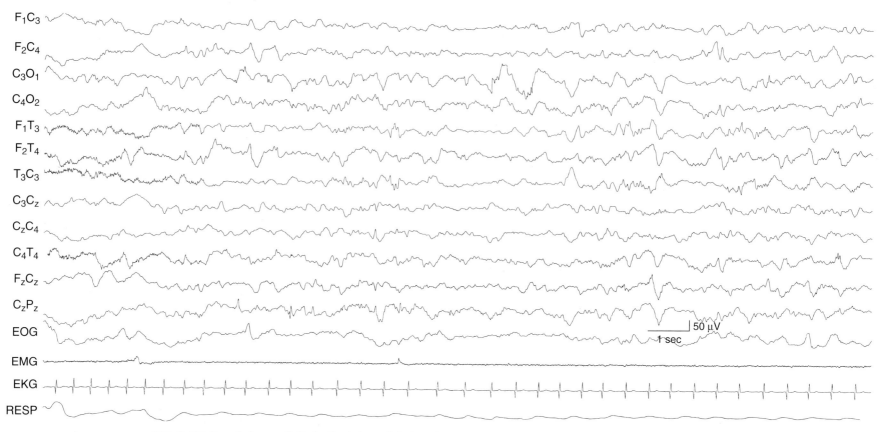

**FIG. 6–32. Focal slow activity in the left occipital region.** Moderate to moderately high voltage, 1- to 3-Hz activity is found in the left occipital region in this term infant with a congenital cystic lesion in that region.

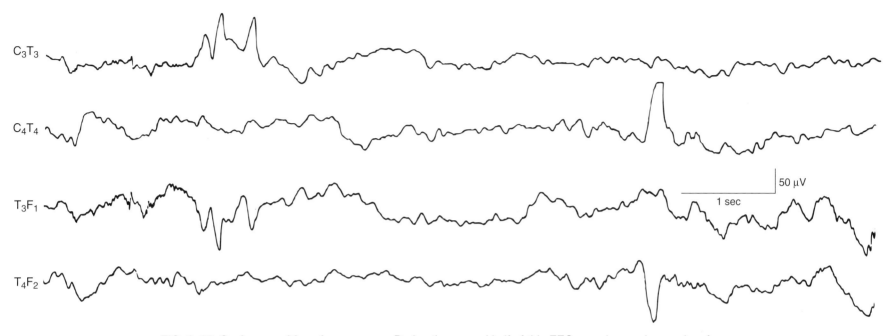

**FIG. 6–33. Surface-positive sharp waves.** During the second half of this EEG sample, an abnormal surface-positive high-voltage sharp wave is seen in the right temporal region. Earlier, moderate-voltage temporal sharp waves are repetitive with both surface-positive and surface-negative components. This sample is selected from a standard 12-channel EEG recording. (From Hrachovy RA, Mizrahi EM, Kellaway P. Electroencephalography of the newborn. In: Daly DD, Pedley TA, eds. *Current practice of clinical electroencephalography,* 2nd ed. New York: Raven Press, 1990:201–241.)

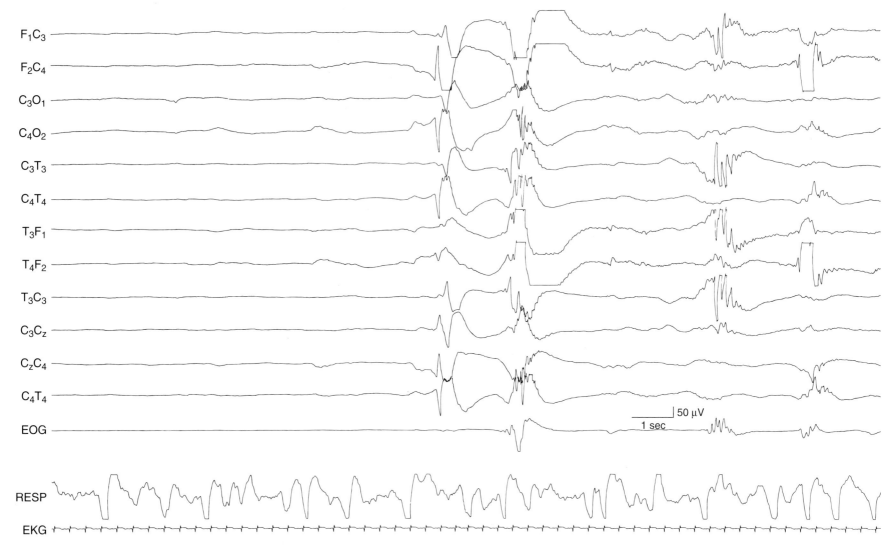

**FIG. 6–34. Surface-positive sharp waves in the premature.** After a period of quiescence, a high-voltage surface-positive sharp wave is present in the right central region. This is followed by abnormal spike and sharp-wave activity a few seconds later. Eventually, a temporal theta burst (a normal feature) is present. This EEG is from a 29- to 30-week CA infant with an intraventricular hemorrhage.

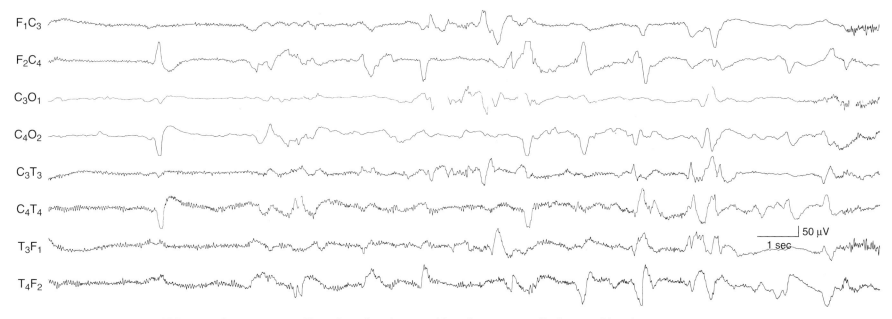

**FIG. 6–35. Occurrence and location of surface-positive sharp waves.** Surface-positive sharp waves may appear as a unilateral, single transient, as in the early portion of this sample, or they may recur at a relatively frequent rate and appear asynchronously on the two sides as in the latter portion of this sample. This sample is taken from the EEG of a 36-week CA infant with intraventricular hemorrhage. The background activity is depressed and undifferentiated; filtered electromyogram artifact is present in the frontal and temporal leads.

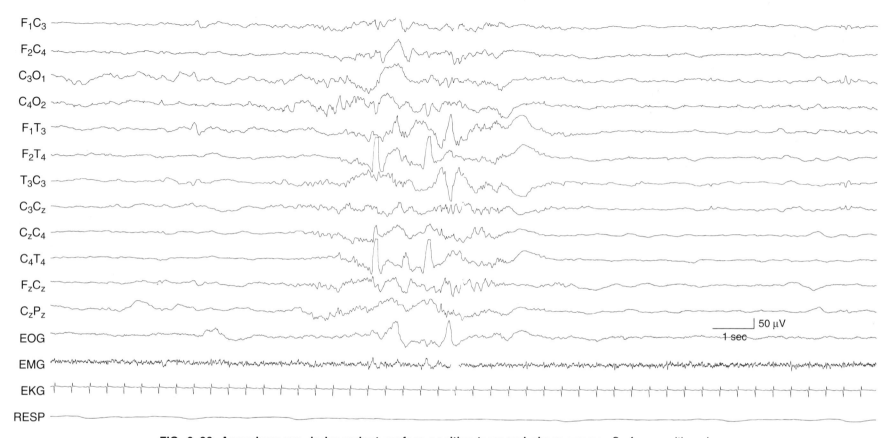

**FIG. 6–36. Asynchronous, independent surface-positive temporal sharp waves.** Surface-positive sharp waves are present independently in the left and right temporal regions in this 35-week CA infant with a chromosomal abnormality, dysmorphic features, and germinal matrix hemorrhage.

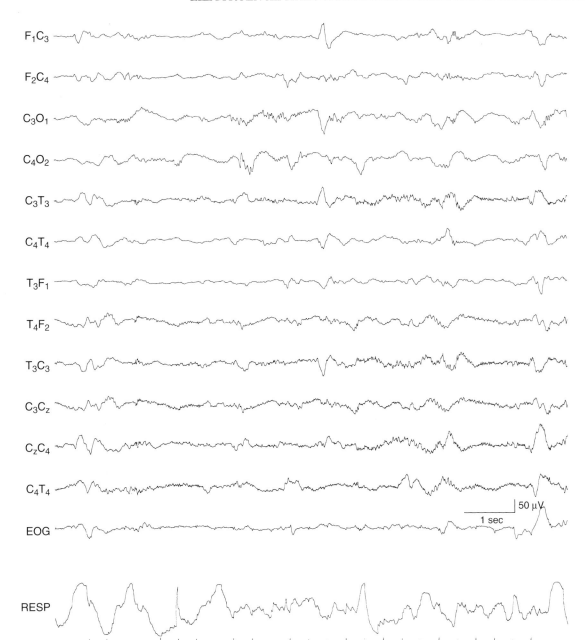

**FIG. 6–37. Surface-positive sharp wave of moderate voltage.** A surface-positive sharp wave of moderate voltage is present in the left central region. The background EEG activity is within the range of normal variation and consistent with a 34- to 35-week CA in this infant with periventricular leukomalacia.

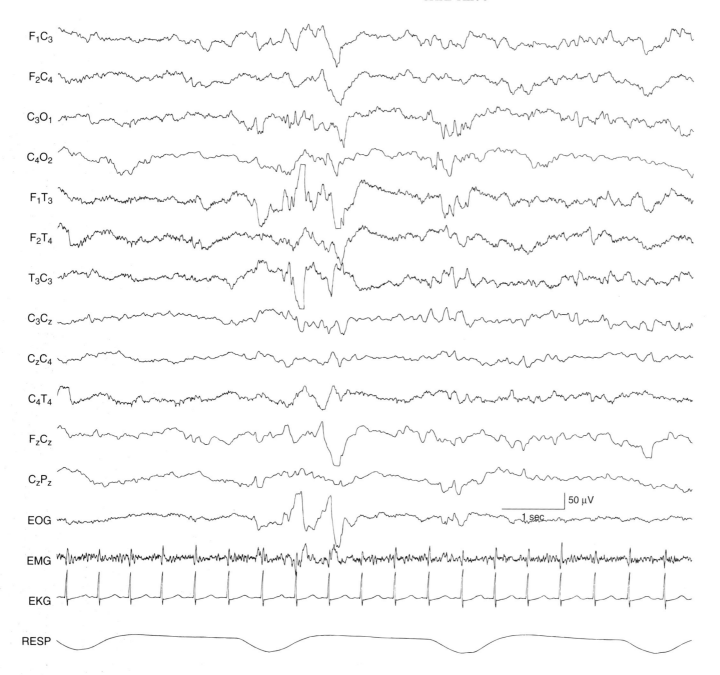

**FIG. 6–38. Surface-positive sharp waves in the temporal region with complex morphology.** A sharp wave with both surface-positive and surface-negative components is present in the left temporal region in this 40-week CA infant with an intracerebral hemorrhage in the left temporal lobe.

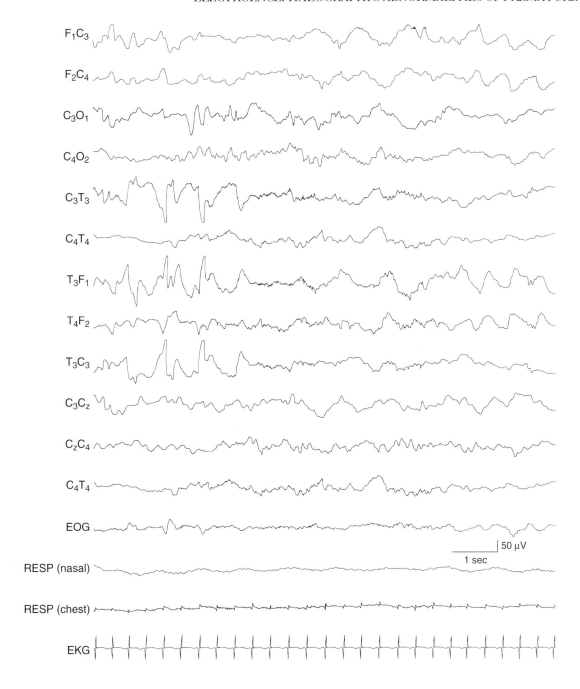

**FIG. 6–39. Temporal sharp waves with complex morphology.** Abnormal temporal sharp waves with complex morphology are present in the left temporal region in the early portion of this sample of a term infant. The background EEG activity is normal and includes some intermittent, rhythmic delta activity in the frontal regions bilaterally. (See Chapter 5 for additional samples of abnormal temporal sharp waves.)

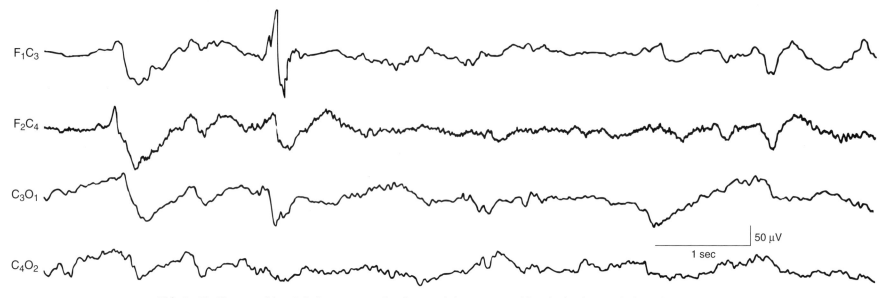

F₁C₃

F₂C₄

C₃O₁

C₄O₂

50 μV

1 sec

**FIG. 6–40. Abnormal frontal sharp wave.** An abnormal sharp wave, with polyphasic morphology, is seen in the left frontal region in this term infant. This is a selected sample from a 12-channel EEG. (From Hrachovy RA, Mizrahi EM, Kellaway P. Electroencephalography of the newborn. In: Daly DD, Pedley TA, eds. *Current practice of clinical electroencephalography,* 2nd ed. New York: Raven Press, 1990:201–241, with permission.)

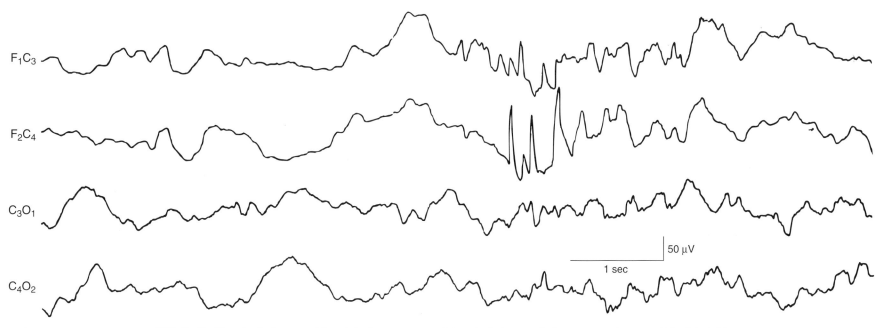

**FIG. 6–41. Burst of abnormal frontal sharp waves.** A burst of abnormal sharp waves is present in the right frontal region in this term infant. This is a selected sample from a 12-channel EEG. (From Hrachovy RA, Mizrahi EM, Kellaway P. Electroencephalography of the newborn. In: Daly DD, Pedley TA, eds. *Current practice of clinical electroencephalography,* 2nd ed. New York: Raven Press, 1990:201–241, with permission.)

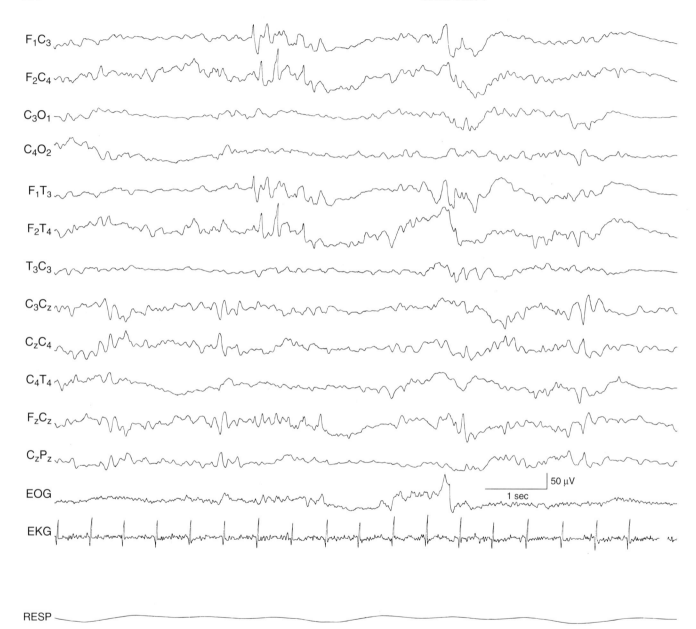

**FIG. 6–42. Independent bilateral abnormal frontal sharp waves.** Abnormal frontal sharp waves are present in the first half of this sample. Frontal sharp transients (an expected developmental milestone in this epoch) are present in the second half of the sample, although abnormal because of their asymmetry. In addition, the background EEG activity is undifferentiated in this 40-week CA infant with lactic acidosis and pulmonary insufficiency.

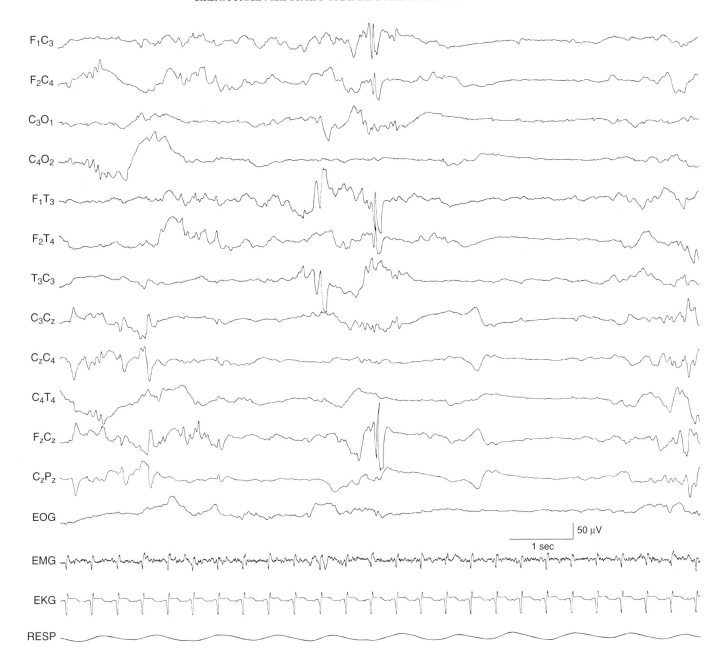

**FIG. 6–43. Bilateral frontal spikes.** High-voltage spikes are present in the frontal regions bilaterally, higher in amplitude on the left and well expressed in the midline frontal region. A temporal sharp wave on the left occurs earlier. The background EEG activity is discontinuous in this 38-week CA infant with cerebral dysgenesis, congenital ventriculomegaly, and choroid plexus hemorrhage.

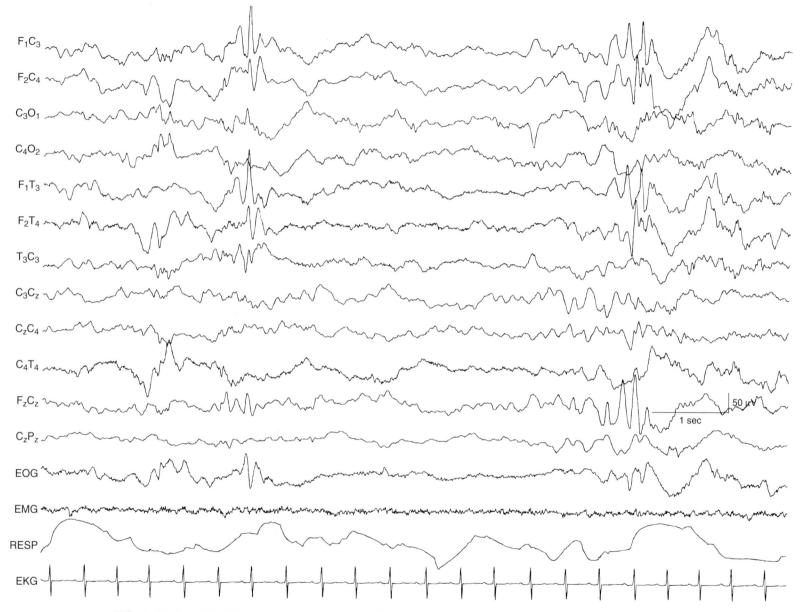

**FIG. 6–44. Bilateral frontal sharp waves.** Intermittently occurring high-voltage sharp waves are seen in the frontal regions bilaterally. The background EEG activity is within the range of normal variation in this 42-week CA infant suspected of having seizures, but without clinical or electrical seizures documented by prolonged EEG.

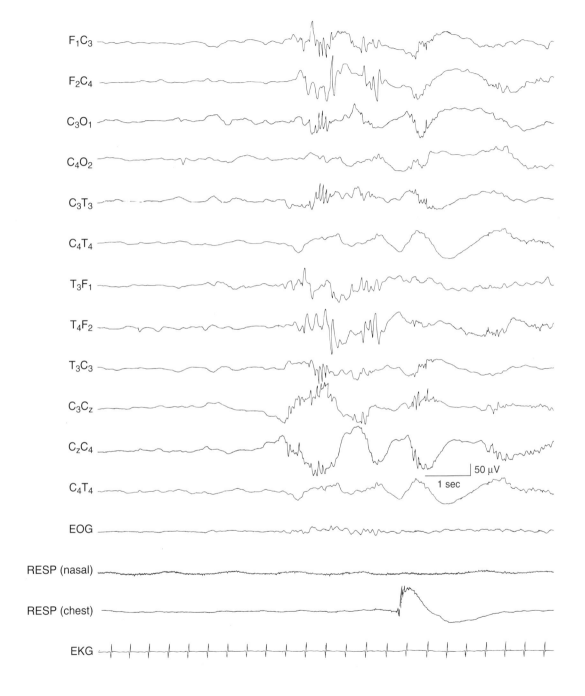

**FIG. 6–45. Frontal sharp waves and independent central spikes.** There are independent high-voltage sharp waves in the right frontal region and runs of low-voltage spikes in the left central region in this 32-week CA infant.

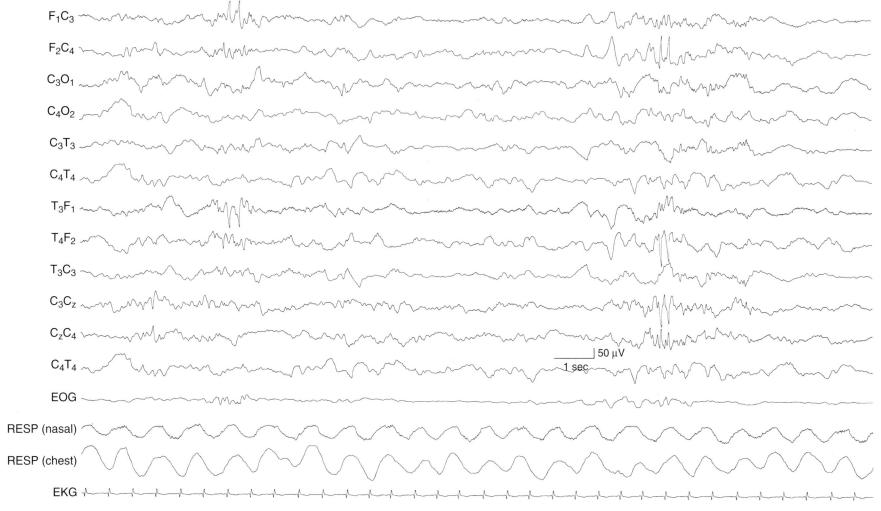

**FIG. 6–46. Midline and lateralized frontal spikes.** Abnormal spikes appear in the left frontal region and, later in the sample, spikes appear in the right frontal region with expression in the midline central region in this term infant.

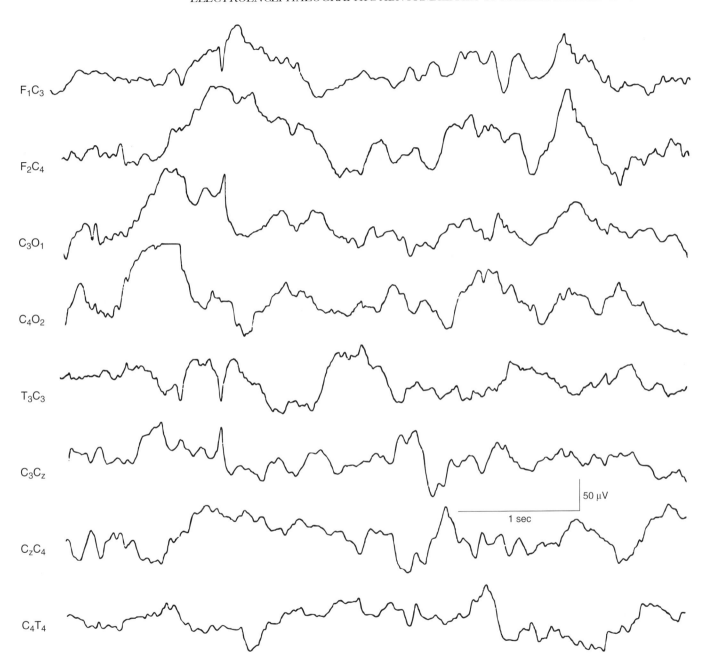

**FIG. 6-47. Central rapid spike.** A single spike discharge is present in the left central region with normal background EEG activity in this term infant. The sample is taken from a 12-channel EEG recording.

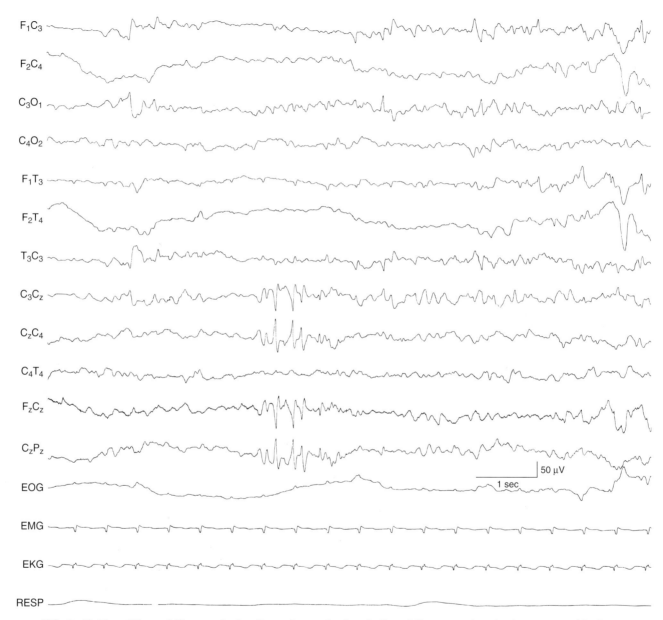

**FIG. 6–48. Repetitive midline central spikes.** A run of spikes in the midline central region is expressed in the Cz electrode in this 38-week CA infant with cardiac failure and grade I intraventricular hemorrhage.

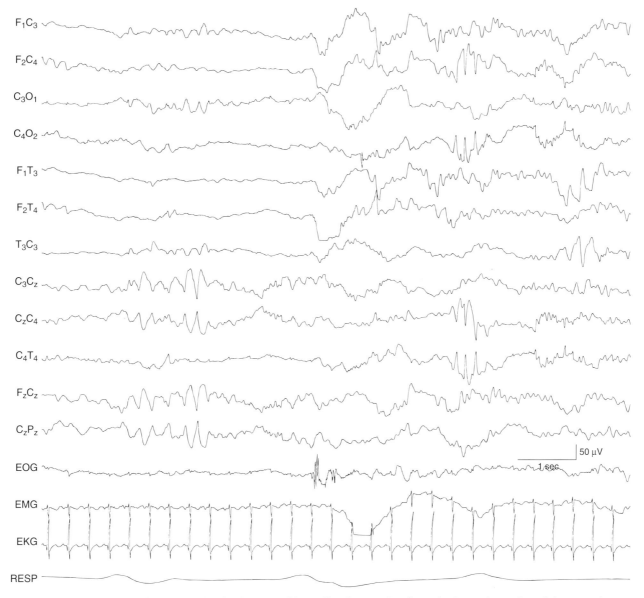

**FIG. 6–49. Central midline, rhythmic theta, and lateralized central spikes.** In the early portion of the recording, rhythmic theta activity appears in the midline central region, and later, a run of rhythmic spikes in the right central region. The infant was born at 28 weeks CA and, at the time of EEG recording, was 35 weeks CA. An acute grade III intraventricular hemorrhage was resolving at the time of EEG recording, although posthemorrhagic hydrocephalus and a porencephalic cyst had extended into the left frontal ventricular horn.

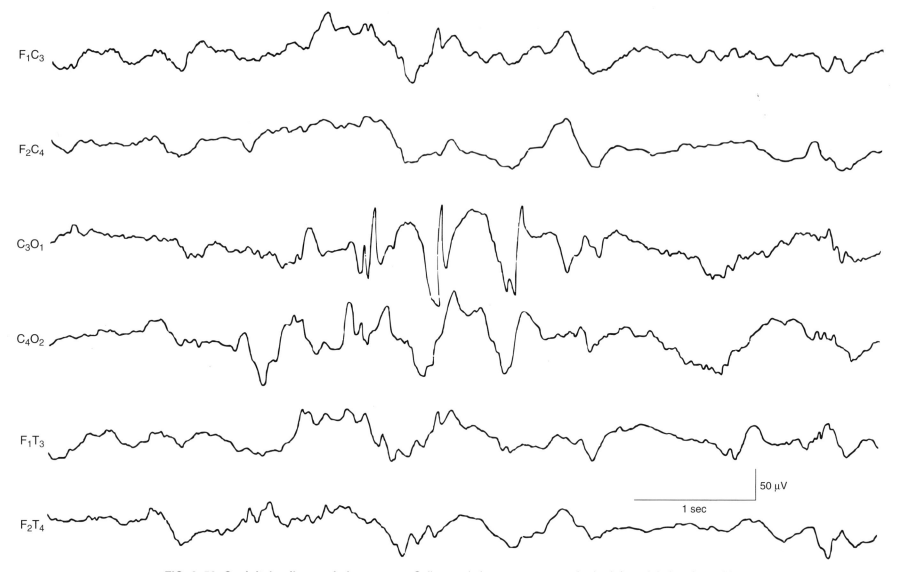

F₁C₃

F₂C₄

C₃O₁

C₄O₂

F₁T₃

50 µV

1 sec

F₂T₄

**FIG. 6–50. Occipital spikes and slow waves.** Spikes and slow waves appear in the left occipital region, with some reflection of the slow-wave component on the right. The background EEG activity is within the range of normal variation in this term infant. This sample is selected from a 12-channel EEG.

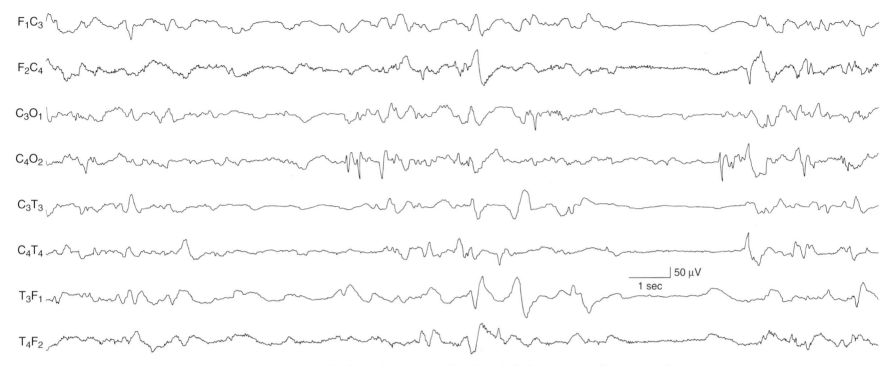

**FIG. 6–51. Occipital spikes and independent temporal and central sharp waves.** Recurrent spikes are seen in the right occipital region early in this sample. Immediately after this burst, frontal sharp transients appear, a normal phenomenon. Then temporal sharp waves on the left are followed by an independent sharp wave on the right.

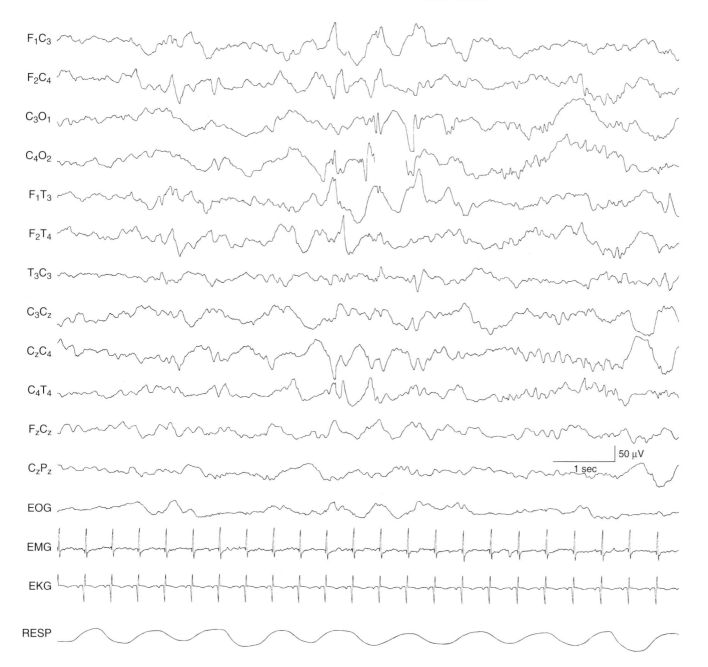

**FIG. 6–52. Bilateral, independent occipital spikes.** Spike and slow-wave complexes are seen independently in the left and right occipital regions in this 40-week CA infant with the peroxisomal disorder, Zellweger syndrome.

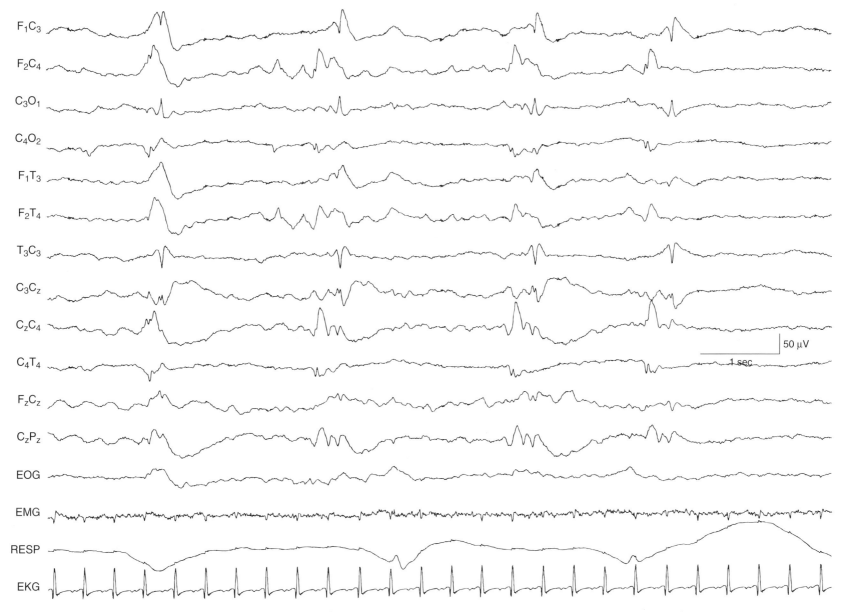

**FIG. 6–53. Multifocal sharp waves.** Sharp waves, with varying morphology, appear independently in the left and right central regions in a semiperiodic manner. The background activity is depressed and undifferentiated in this 44-week CA infant with the inborn error of metabolism, ornithine carbamylase transferase deficiency.

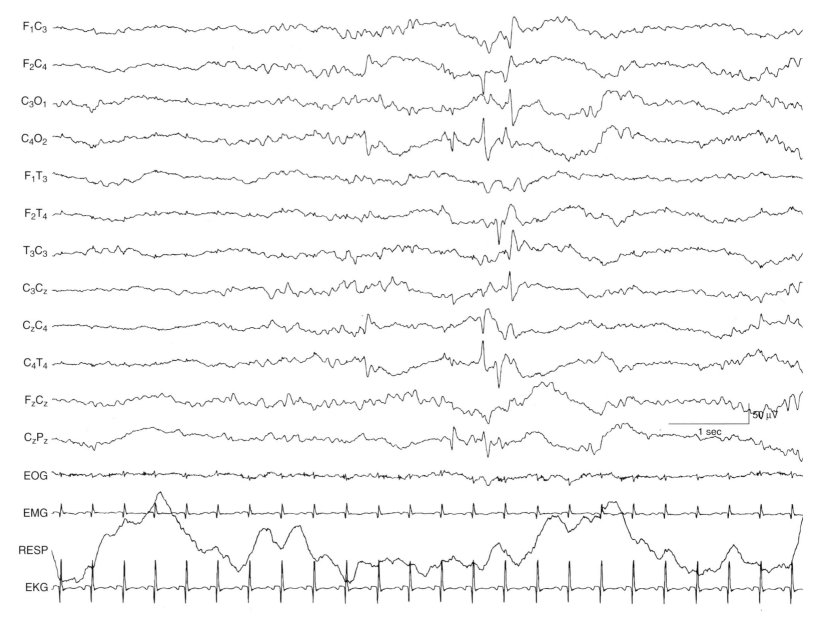

**FIG. 6–54. Multifocal spikes and sharp waves.** Spikes and sharp waves appear independently in the left and right central and right temporal regions. The background EEG activity is undifferentiated in this 40-week CA infant with congenital heart disease.

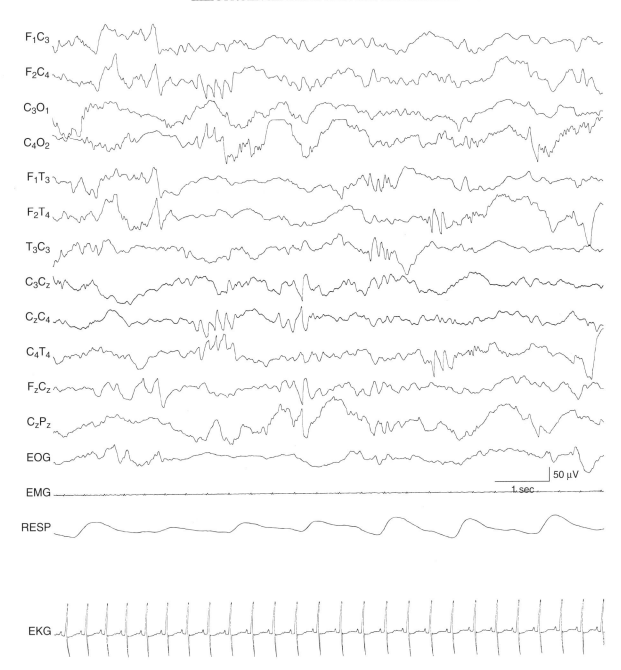

**FIG. 6–55. Multifocal sharp waves with rhythmic morphology.** Very brief bursts of rhythmic sharp theta activity appear independently in the left central and left and right temporal regions. The background activity is undifferentiated in this infant with laboratory confirmed herpes simplex encephalitis.

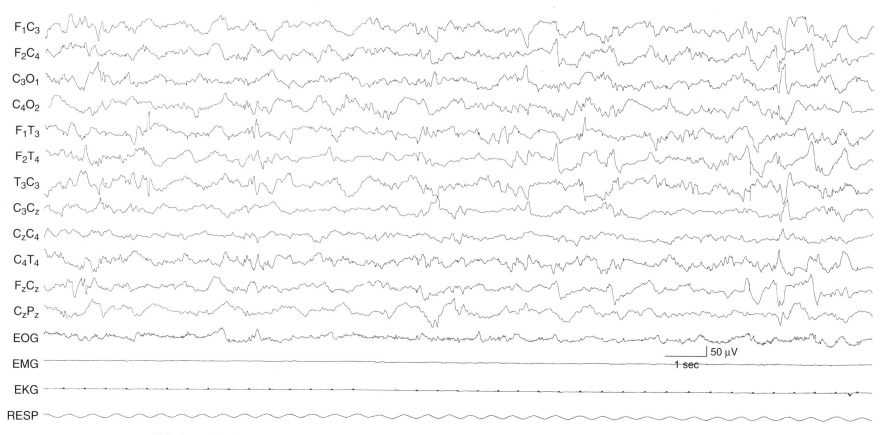

**FIG. 6–56. Surface-positive and surface-negative multifocal sharp waves.** Sharp waves are present in the left and right central, left and right temporal, and right frontal regions. Some of the waveforms are surface positive (left temporal early in the sample), and others are surface negative in this term infant with renal failure.

# CHAPTER 7

# Neonatal Seizures

The electrographic and clinical characteristics of seizures in the neonate are unique compared with those of older children and adults. In the neonate, interictal epileptiform discharges are rarely present to aid in diagnosis, electrographic seizure patterns vary widely, electrical seizure activity does not always accompany all behaviors currently considered to be seizures, and electrical seizure activity may occur without evident clinical seizures (Kellaway and Hrachovy, 1983; Mizrahi and Kellaway, 1987; Mizrahi and Kellaway, 1998).

This chapter addresses the electroencephalographic (EEG) and clinical features of neonatal seizures. Other pertinent issues concerning neonatal seizures that relate to epileptogenesis of the immature brain, the effect of seizures on the developing brain, pathophysiology, etiology, therapy, and prognosis are beyond the scope of an atlas of neonatal electroencephalography, but are considered in detail elsewhere (Bye et al., 1997; Clancy, 1996; Holmes, 2002; Lombroso, 1996a, 1996b; Mizrahi, 1999, 2001; Mizrahi and Clancy, 2000; Mizrahi and Kellaway, 1998; Mizrahi and Watanabe, 2002; Painter et al., 1999; Rennie, 1997; Scher, 1997, 2002; Stafstrom and Holmes, 2002; Swann, 2002; Swann and Hablitz, 2000; Tharp, 2002; Velisek and Moshe, 2002).

In considering neonatal seizures, important features of interpretation include recognition of EEG seizures and the determination of the significance of focal sharp waves that may occur between seizures. Electrical seizure activity in the newborn has some features similar to those of older children and adults, but also several features characteristic of the neonate. These are discussed later. As previously discussed in Chapters 4 through 6, focal sharp waves in the neonatal EEG may be normal, of uncertain diagnostic significance, or abnormal. However, they generally do not correlate with the presence of epileptic seizures. Thus the finding of isolated sharp waves in an infant suspected of having had a seizure does not provide evidence that a seizure has occurred or will occur.

In addition, the correlation of electrical seizure activity with the occurrence of clinical seizures is critical. This is most effectively accomplished by direct observation at the bedside during EEG recording or by EEG-video monitoring. When the clinical behaviors in question are not witnessed directly or recorded on video, the neurophysiologist must rely on the description of the clinical event through notations made by the electroneurodiagnostic technologist (ENDT) at the time of recording.

## CLINICAL CHARACTERISTICS OF NEONATAL SEIZURES

The occurrence of clinical seizures in neonates may often be the first, and sometimes the only, manifestation of central nervous system (CNS) dysfunction. As such, seizure occurrence represents an emergent problem since causes of seizures can be successfully treated, with the potential to limit associated brain injury. Direct or indirect alterations may occur in respiration, heart rate, or systemic blood pressure in association with seizures or their aggressive therapy. Traditionally, it has been believed that seizures in the developing brain do not cause further brain injury beyond that caused by seizure etiology. Although more recent data continue to suggest that the immature brain is more resistant to seizure-induced injury than is the mature brain (Albala et al., 1984; Sperber et al., 1991; Stafstrom et al., 1992; Thurber et al., 1994), recent animal studies also suggest that long-term consequences may result from seizures in the developing brain in terms of disturbances of learning, memory, or behavior (Cilio et al., 2003; de Rogalski et al., 2001;

Holmes and Ben-Ari, 2001; Holmes et al., 2002; Villeneuve et al., 2000), although this still remains controversial.

The concepts of which motor and autonomic phenomena constitute clinical seizures have continually changed over the years (Burke, 1954; Cadilhac et al., 1959; Dreyfus-Brisac and Monod, 1964; Fenichel et al., 1979; Harris and Tizard, 1960; Kellaway and Hrachovy, 1983; Minkowski et al., 1955; Mizrahi and Kellaway, 1987; Perlman and Volpe, 1983; Rose and Lombroso, 1970; Volpe, 1973, 1989; Watanabe et al., 1977). More recently, greater consensus has occurred. All of the clinical behaviors currently considered neonatal seizures have been recorded and analyzed, using EEG/polygraphic/video monitoring (Biagioni et al., 1998; Bye and Flanagan, 1995; Mizrahi and Kellaway, 1987; Plouin, 2000; Scher et al., 1993). Some behaviors are not consistently accompanied by electrical seizure activity, and many consistently occur without ictal discharges (Mizrahi and Kellaway, 1987). Despite this variable relation of clinical seizures to electrical seizure activity, all clinical seizures occur in association with CNS disorders. These findings indicate that different types of neonatal seizures may reflect different pathophysiologic mechanisms—epileptic or nonepileptic—and regardless of their pathophysiology and relation to electrical seizure activity, the clinical behaviors known as neonatal seizures reliably indicate the presence of CNS dysfunction.

## TERMINOLOGY AND CLASSIFICATION

### Electroclinical Classification
Although the pathophysiologic mechanisms underlying neonatal seizures may still be debated, it is important to develop a working seizure-classification system that can be effectively used to identify specific abnormal clinical behaviors associated with CNS disease. Regardless of their pathophysiology, all of the phenomena considered to be seizures are "seizures" in the generic sense, without necessarily implying that they are all epileptic. Eventually it may become evident that some "seizures" are epileptic in origin, whereas others are initiated and elaborated by nonepileptic mechanisms.

A number of approaches are used in the classification of clinical neonatal seizures. A classification system based on the relation of EEG seizure patterns to clinical events is presented in **Table 7–1** along with other clinical and electrographic signs that may aid in diagnosis (Kellaway and Mizrahi, 1987; Mizrahi and Kellaway, 1987). **Table 7–2** lists seizure types, clinical features, electrographic

**TABLE 7–1.** *Classification of neonatal seizures based on electroclinical findings*

**Clinical seizures with a consistent electrocortical correlate**
(Pathophysiology: epileptic)
Focal clonic
    Unifocal
    Multifocal
    Hemiconvulsive
    Axial
Focal tonic
    Asymmetric truncal posturing
    Limb posturing
    Sustained eye deviation
Myoclonic
    Generalized
    Focal
Spasms
    Flexor
    Extensor
    Mixed extensor/flexor

**Clinical seizures without a consistent electrocortical correlate**
(Pathophysiology: presumed nonepileptic)
Myoclonic
    Generalized
    Focal
    Fragmentary
Generalized tonic
    Flexor
    Extensor
    Mixed extensor/flexor
Motor automatisms
    Oral–buccal–lingual movements
    Ocular signs
    Progression movements
    Complex purposeless movements

**Electrical seizures without clinical seizure activity**

From Mizrahi EM, Kellaway P. *Diagnosis and management of neonatal seizures.* Philadelphia: Lippincott-Raven, 1998.

correlates, and presumed pathophysiology. In addition, from the perspective of the neonatal EEG, neonatal seizures can be classified according to the temporal relation between the electrical event and the clinical event: electroclinical, clinical-only, and electrical-only seizures.

**TABLE 7–2.** *Clinical characteristics, classification, and presumed pathophysiology of neonatal seizures*

| Classification | Characterization |
|---|---|
| Focal clonic | Repetitive, rhythmic contractions of muscle groups of the limbs, face, or trunk<br>May be unifocal or multifocal<br>May occur synchronously or asynchronously in muscle groups on one side of the body<br>May occur simultaneously, but asynchronously on both sides<br>Cannot be suppressed by restraint<br>Pathophysiology: epileptic |
| Focal tonic | Sustained posturing of single limbs<br>Sustained asymmetric posturing of the trunk<br>Sustained eye deviation<br>Cannot be provoked by stimulation or suppressed by restraint<br>Pathophysiology: epileptic |
| Generalized tonic | Sustained symmetric posturing of limbs, trunk, and neck<br>May be flexor, extensor, or mixed extensor/flexor<br>May be provoked or intensified by stimulation<br>May be suppressed by restraint or repositioning<br>Presumed pathophysiology: nonepileptic |
| Myoclonic | Random, single, rapid contractions of muscle groups of the limbs, face, or trunk<br>Typically not repetitive or may recur at a slow rate<br>May be generalized, focal, or fragmentary<br>May be provoked by stimulation<br>Presumed pathophysiology: may be epileptic or nonepileptic |
| Spasms | May be flexor, extensor, or mixed extensor/flexor<br>May occur in clusters<br>Cannot be provoked by stimulation or suppressed by restraint<br>Pathophysiology: epileptic |
| Motor automatisms<br>  Ocular signs | Random and roving eye movements or nystagmus (distinct from tonic eye deviation)<br>May be provoked or intensified by tactile stimulation<br>Presumed pathophysiology: nonepileptic |
|   Oral–buccal–lingual movements | Sucking, chewing, tongue protrusions<br>May be provoked or intensified by stimulation<br>Presumed pathophysiology: nonepileptic |
|   Progression movements | Rowing or swimming movements<br>Pedaling or bicycling movements of the legs<br>May be provoked or intensified by stimulation<br>May be suppressed by restraint or repositioning<br>Presumed pathophysiology: nonepileptic |
|   Complex purposeless movements | Sudden arousal with transient increased random activity of limbs<br>May be provoked or intensified by stimulation<br>Presumed pathophysiology: nonepileptic |

From Mizrahi EM, Kellaway P. *Diagnosis and management of neonatal seizures.* Philadelphia: Lippincott-Raven, 1998, with permission.

### Electroclinical Seizures

Electroclinical seizures are characterized by a temporal overlap between clinical seizures and electrical seizure activity on EEG. In many instances, the electrical and clinical events are closely associated, with the onset and termination of both events coinciding. However, this may not always be the case: clinical onset may precede electrical onset, electrical onset may precede clinical onset, and either the clinical or electrical seizure may terminate first.

Focal clonic, focal tonic, and some myoclonic seizures and spasms are associated with electrical seizure activity. Some clinical features of focal clonic seizures are unique to this age group. The seizures may be multifocal with alternating, asynchronous, or migrating clonic jerking; hemiconvulsive, involving an entire side of the body; or may appear as clonic jerking of axial musculature of trunk, abdomen, neck, or tongue. Focal tonic seizures with asymmetric trunk or limb posturing or tonic eye deviation also are associated with electrical seizure activity. In addition, some focal or generalized myoclonic jerks also are consistently accompanied by EEG seizure discharges. A special, and rare, circumstance is the occurrence of spasms associated with generalized voltage attenuation or generalized slow sharp transients.

Focal clonic seizures most often occur in infants who appear to be awake and alert. Typically, the background EEG activity is normal. The etiologic factors are most often cerebral infarction, intracerebral hemorrhage, subarachnoid hemorrhage, and, more rarely, metabolic disorders such as hypoglycemia and hypocalcemia. The short-term outcome of infants with focal clonic seizures is good compared with that of infants who have other types of seizures.

### Clinical-Only Seizures

Some types of clinical seizures have no specific relation to electrical seizure activity. Those that occur in the absence of any electrical seizure activity include generalized tonic posturing, motor automatisms, and some myoclonic seizures. Generalized tonic posturing may be flexor or extensor or may be mixed extensor/flexor. Motor automatisms include oral–buccal–lingual movements such as lip-smacking, sucking, and tongue protrusion; ocular signs such as roving eye movements, blinking, and nystagmus; progression movements such as pedaling or stepping of legs, or swimming or rotary movements of the arms; and complex purposeless movements such as struggling or thrashing. These clinical events, referred to as "motor automatisms" (Mizrahi and Kellaway, 1987) are equivalent to some described as "little peripheral phenomena" or "anarchic" by Dreyfus-Brisac and Monod (1964); as "subtle seizures" by Volpe (1973); and as "minimal seizures" by Lombroso (1974). Myoclonic jerks also may be present without accompanying EEG seizure discharges. They may be generalized, or they may be confined to limited muscle groups.

Tonic posturing, motor automatisms, and myoclonic jerks most often occur in infants who are lethargic or obtunded. The EEG background activity is typically depressed and undifferentiated. In some infants with these types of seizures, recordings have shown no electrical activity of cerebral origin. The etiology of these seizure types is most often hypoxic–ischemic encephalopathy. Compared with focal clonic and focal tonic seizures, seizures unassociated with electrical seizure activity indicate a poorer prognosis, with high morbidity and mortality.

### Electrical Seizure Activity without Evident Clinical Seizures

Subclinical electrical seizure activity—that is, electrical seizure activity with no clinical accompaniment (Clancy et al., 1988; Mizrahi and Kellaway, 1987)—occurs in several situations. This may occur in an infant who is pharmacologically paralyzed for respiratory care. Typically no behavioral changes are associated with seizure discharges of the depressed brain or alpha seizure discharges (see later). Third, antiepileptic drugs (AEDs) may suppress the clinical component of an electroclinical seizure but not the electrical component; the clinical seizure may be controlled, but electrical seizure activity may persist.

## Additional Issues of Classification

### Seizures That Are Predominantly Autonomic

It has been reported that some clinical seizures consist predominantly of changes in respiration, blood pressure, or heart rate; pupillary constriction or dilatation; pallor or flushing; or drooling or salivation (Mizrahi and Kellaway, 1998). The relation of these paroxysmal autonomic events to electrical seizure activity has not been firmly established, nor has the frequency of their occurrence as ictal phenomena. For example, apnea can occur as an ictal event with associated electrical seizure activity, but this is rare compared with other causes of apnea in newborns. If apnea occurs in close relation to an EEG seizure discharge, it is likely to be accompanied by other clinical seizure phenomena. Thus these autonomic features more likely occur as components of clinical seizures with motor manifestations than as the sole manifestation of a clinical seizure.

## Mixed Seizure Types

Several types of seizures may occur in the same infant: electroclinical, clinical only, and electrical only. For example, an infant with tonic posturing unassociated with electrical seizure activity also may exhibit focal clonic seizures that have a distinct electrical signature. In addition, electrical seizure activity may occur without behavioral correlates in infants who at other times have clinical seizures.

## Epileptic Syndromes

Few well-defined epileptic syndromes are found in the neonate (Commission, 1989; Mizrahi and Clancy, 2000); two are benign, and two are catastrophic. The benign syndromes are benign neonatal convulsions and benign familial neonatal convulsions. These are characterized by focal clonic or focal tonic seizures that are electroclinical, have normal-background EEG activity, and typically have a good outcome (Plouin and Anderson, 2002).

Some neonatal seizures are considered idiopathic because no cause can be identified, and no long-term sequelae ensue. Many of these infants are thought to have benign neonatal convulsions, more recently referred to as benign idiopathic neonatal seizures (Plouin, 1990, 1992; Plouin and Anderson, 2002). The infants are typically term and products of normal pregnancy and delivery. The seizures are usually brief, most often clonic, and have their onset between days 4 and 6 of life. Dehan et al. (1977) described an interictal background EEG pattern that may be present in these infants, *theta pointu alternant,* although it is not considered specific to this disorder (Navelet et al., 1981; Plouin and Anderson, 2002) (see later).

Benign familial neonatal convulsions have a pattern of autosomal transmission based on a locus on chromosome 20 (Leppert et al., 1989; Quattlebaum et al., 1979). Singh and colleagues (1998) identified a submicroscopic deletion of chromosome 20q13.3 and encoded a novel voltage-gated potassium channel, KCNQ2, as the basis of this disorder. This disorder is now considered to be one of several epileptic disorders characterized as a channelopathy (Noebels, 2001; Leppert, 2001). Benign familial neonatal convulsions had been considered to be benign because initial reports suggested no long-term neurologic sequelae. However, subsequent studies indicate that not all affected infants have normal outcomes (Ronen et al., 1993).

The catastrophic syndromes are early myoclonic encephalopathy (EME) (Aicardi and Goutieres, 1978; Aicardi, 1992) and early infantile epileptic encephalopathy (EIEE) (Ohtahara et al., 1976; Ohtahara et al., 1992). The catastrophic syndromes are compared in **Table 7–3** and recently were reviewed by Aicardi and Ohtahara (2002).

**TABLE 7–3.** *Comparison of early myoclonic encephalopathy (EME) and early infantile epileptic encephalopathy (EIEE)*

| | EME | EIEE |
|---|---|---|
| Age at onset | Neonatal period | Within first 3 mo |
| Neurologic status at onset | Abnormal at birth or at seizure onset | Always abnormal, even before seizure onset |
| Characteristic seizure type | Erratic or fragmentary myoclonus | Tonic spasms (early) |
| Additional seizure type | Massive myoclonus<br>Partial seizures<br>Tonic spasms (late) | Partial seizures<br>Massive myoclonus (rare) |
| Background EEG | Suppression burst | Suppression burst |
| Etiology | Inborn errors of metabolism<br>Familial<br>Cryptogenic | Cerebral dysgenesis<br>Anoxia<br>Cryptogenic |
| Natural course | Progressive impairment | Static impairment |
| Incidence of death | Very high, occurring in infancy | High, occurring in infancy, childhood, or adolescence |
| Status of survivors | Vegetative state | Severe mental retardation<br>Quadriplegia and bedridden status |
| Long-term seizure or syndrome evolution | Tonic spasms | West syndrome<br>Lennox–Gastaut syndrome |

From Mizrahi EM, Clancy RR. Neonatal seizures: Early-onset seizure syndromes and their consequences for development. *Ment Retard Dev Disabil Res Rev* 2000;6:240–241, with permission; based on data from Aicardi J, Ohtahara S. Severe neonatal epilepsies with suppression-burst pattern. In: Roger J, Bureau M, Dravet C, et al., eds. *Epileptic syndromes in infancy, childhood, and adolescence,* 3rd ed. London: John Libbey, 2002:33–44.

## INTERICTAL ELECTROENCEPHALOGRAPHIC FEATURES

### Focal Sharp Waves

In older children and adults, a focal sharp wave or spike that may appear between electrical seizures typically indicates the potential for an electrical seizure to arise from that region. However, in the neonate, interictal epileptiform discharges are rarely present to aid in diagnosis. Despite this caveat, isolated sharp waves may arise in the same region of eventual electrical seizure onset, and in these exceptional instances, they are considered epileptiform (**Fig. 7–1**). However, focal sharp waves in the neonate typically are not considered evidence of a focal epileptogenic brain abnormality and therefore provide no useful information concerning the presence or absence of the potential for electrical or clinical seizures in a given infant. Focal sharp waves are discussed in detail in Chapters 5 and 6.

## Background EEG Activity

The features of the background activity in infants suspected of having seizures may be helpful in diagnosis. The character of the background activity will provide information concerning the degree, if any, of brain injury and will provide the basis for consideration of possible diagnoses and prognosis (Bye et al., 1997; McBride et al., 2000; Ortibus et al., 1996). When recording infants suspected of having seizures, those with an abnormal background EEG are more likely eventually to have electroclinical seizures than are those with a normal background (Laroia et al., 1998). In neonates with documented clinical seizures, the degree of abnormality of the background activity may be associated with various seizure types: normal EEG background activity is more closely associated with electroclinical seizures, and abnormal background EEG activity is more closely associated with either clinical-only seizures (Mizrahi and Kellaway, 1987) or electrical-only seizures (Mizrahi and Kellaway, 1987; Pinto and Giliberti, 2001). The character of the background activity also may be helpful in the diagnosis of specific epileptic syndromes. The syndromes of EME and EIEE are associated with a suppression-burst pattern (Aicardi, 1992; Ohtahara, 1992). The background EEG activity of some infants with benign neonatal convulsions has been described as a *theta pointu alternant* pattern (Dehan et al., 1977), although it is not considered specific for the disorder (Navalet et al., 1981; Plouin and Anderson, 2002). This pattern is characterized by generalized theta activity that is occasionally associated with sharp waves. This activity is frequently asynchronous on the sides and occurs discontinuously or in a pattern that alternates with periods of generalized voltage attenuation. The pattern can be present during wakefulness and all stages of sleep. *Theta pointu alternant* may be present for several days after seizures have resolved. However, it can be associated with well-defined etiologies as well as the syndrome of benign neonatal convulsions.

## Ictal EEG Features

Electrical seizure activity consists of sustained rhythmic activity with various morphologies, amplitudes, and frequencies. Electrical seizures are often characterized in terms of their evolution of appearance. The minimal duration of a discharge to be considered an electrical seizure has been defined as 10 seconds (Clancy and Legido, 1987), although this is admittedly arbitrary, and discharges of similar appearance but slightly shorter duration may have the same significance as those of 10 seconds (Oliveira et al., 2000) (**Fig. 7–2**).

Electrical seizure activity is rare before the age of 34 to 35 weeks CA. The precise CA at which the immature brain can consistently initiate and sustain electrical seizure activity has not been defined and may occur only rarely in the premature infant (**Fig. 7–3**). With increasing age, however, electrical seizure activity becomes more frequent and of longer duration (Scher et al., 1993).

All electrical seizure activity in the neonate begins focally, except for the generalized activity associated with some types of myoclonic jerks or with infantile spasms. The region of cortical involvement of the electrical seizure activity will determine the motor manifestations of the clinical seizures. The rate of repetition of the discharge will determine the rate of focal myoclonic and focal clonic activity: slower discharges are associated with slow myoclonic movements (**Fig. 7–4**); faster repetitive discharges are associated with sustained clonic activity (**Fig. 7–5**); and at times, fastest repetitive discharges are associated with focal tonic activity. Muscle group involvement also will determine clinical manifestations. Smaller muscle groups, with smaller degrees of excursion, may move more quickly in response to rhythmic discharges than do larger muscle groups.

### Site of Onset

Electrical seizure activity in the neonate most often arises in the central (**Fig. 7–5**) or temporal region (**Fig. 7–6**) of one hemisphere or the midline central region (**Fig. 7–7**). Less common sites of onset are occipital (**Fig. 7–8**) and frontal regions (**Fig. 7–9**).

### Focality

Most often, in an individual infant, electrical seizure activity is unifocal—always arising from the same brain region. Seizures also may arise from more than one focal area so that, for example, the electrical seizures may arise from different foci at different times. They also may arise from two or more foci at the same time, but with the two foci firing asynchronously (**Figs. 7–10 to 7–12**).

### Frequency, Voltage, and Morphology

Frequency, voltage, and morphology may vary greatly within the same electrical seizure or from one seizure to the next in a given infant. The predominant frequency in a given seizure can be in the alpha, theta, beta, or delta ranges, or a mixture of these. The voltages of the activity also may vary, from extremely low (usually when faster frequencies are present) to very high (commonly seen when slow frequencies are present). The morphology of the electrical activity also may vary, consisting only of spikes of various durations, sharp waves, slow waves, or combinations of the waveforms within a given seizure. Examples of the variability of frequency, voltage, and morphology are shown in **Figs. 7–13 to 7–18**.

### Involvement of Specific Brain Regions

An individual electrical seizure, once begun, may be confined to a specific region (**Fig. 7–19**), or it may spread to involve other regions (**Fig. 7–20**). Spread may be by a gradual widening of the focal area; by abrupt change from a small regional focus to involvement of the entire hemisphere; by migration of the electrical seizure from one area of a hemisphere to another (either in a jacksonian, but most often, in a nonjacksonian fashion); or from one hemisphere to the other.

### Evolution of the Discharge

Some electrical seizure activity may begin abruptly with similar frequencies, voltages, and morphology that remain fairly constant throughout the seizure. However, more often, seizures undergo an evolution in appearance with their character changing throughout its course (**Figs. 7–21 and 7–22**). The changing character throughout an electrical seizure helps in differentiating other nonepileptic rhythmic activity or artifacts from electrical seizure activity.

### Special Ictal Patterns

Some unique ictal patterns occur in neonates with severe encephalopathies: electrical "seizures of the depressed brain" and "alpha seizure discharges." Electrical seizures of the depressed brain are seen in neonates whose background EEG activity is depressed and undifferentiated (**Fig. 7–23**). The discharges are typically low in voltage, long in duration, highly localized, may be unifocal or multifocal, and show little tendency to spread or otherwise change (Kellaway and Hrachovy, 1983). This seizure pattern typically is not accompanied by clinical seizure activity. The presence of this pattern suggests a poor prognosis.

The sudden but transient appearance of rhythmic activity in the alpha frequency band is referred to as alpha seizure activity (Knauss and Carlson, 1978; Willis and Gould, 1980; Watanabe et al., 1982) (**Figs. 7–24 and 7–25**). This pattern is characterized by the sudden appearance of rhythmic 8- to 12-Hz, 20- to 70-$\mu$V activity typically in one temporal or central region; however, it also can evolve from activity that is more clearly epileptic. In addition, it may occur simultaneously, but asynchronously with other electrical seizure activity (**Fig. 7–26**). Its presence is indicative of a severe encephalopathy and suggests a poor prognosis. This pattern also may be present in the absence of any clinical seizures. The paroxysmal alpha pattern should be differentiated from virtually continuous rhythmic, low-voltage activity that is a rare finding in the neonate associated with disorders such as congenital heart disease, chromosomal abnormalities, and administration of CNS active drugs (see Chapter 6) (Hrachovy and O'Donnell, 1996).

### Generalized Electrical Seizure Patterns

Electrographic events that are considered generalized seizure patterns are rare in the neonate and are associated with only a few specific clinical seizure types. Generalized sharp transients may be associated with generalized myoclonus (**Fig. 7–27**). Spasms may occur in association with generalized voltage attenuation (**Fig. 7–28**) or generalized sharp transients.

### Electrical Seizure Activity and Medication Effects

The most important effect medication may have on electroclinical seizures is the elimination of clinical seizures while electrical seizures persist. In addition to the occurrence of both electrical seizure activity of the depressed brain and the paroxysmal alpha pattern (e.g., alpha seizure pattern) discussed earlier, electrical seizure activity without clinical seizures may be present in infants treated with AEDs and in those treated with pharmacologic paralytic agents.

A common situation occurs during the short-term administration of AEDs in an infant with electroclinical seizures. This may result first in control of the clinical seizures with persistence of the electrical seizure (**Fig. 7–29**). The phenomenon has been termed "decoupling" of the clinical from the electrical seizure (Mizrahi and Kellaway, 1987). After continued AED administration, the electrical seizure activity may become modulated and may eventually be eliminated. However, frequently increasing AED dosage or additional agents may not completely eliminate electrical seizure discharges. In instances in which electrical seizures are controlled, they may recur without clinical accompaniment.

Another circumstance in which electrical seizures occur without clinical seizures because of pharmacologic therapy is when infants are paralyzed for respiratory ventilation and other medical reasons. Obviously, an infant who is paralyzed cannot manifest motor signs of seizures.

**LIST OF FIGURES**

**FIGURES CONTINUE ON THE NEXT PAGE**

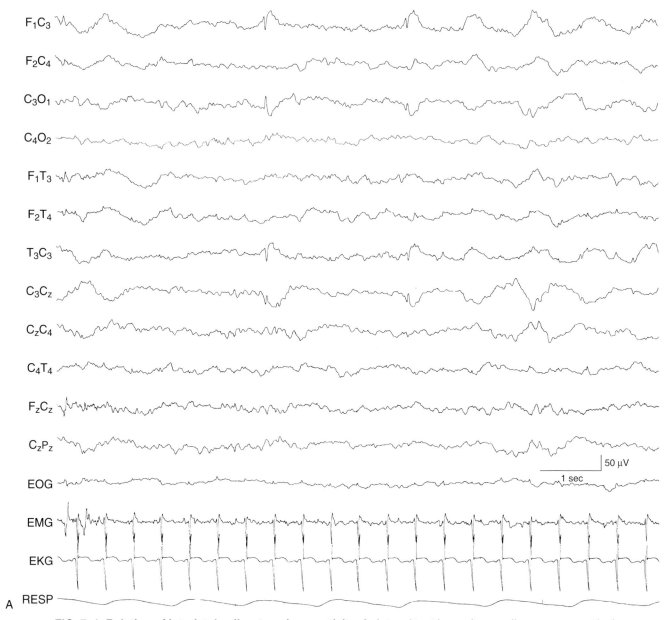

**FIG. 7–1. Relation of interictal spikes to seizure activity. A:** Intermittent low-voltage spikes are present in the left central region; their occurrence waxed and waned in other portions of the recording (not shown).

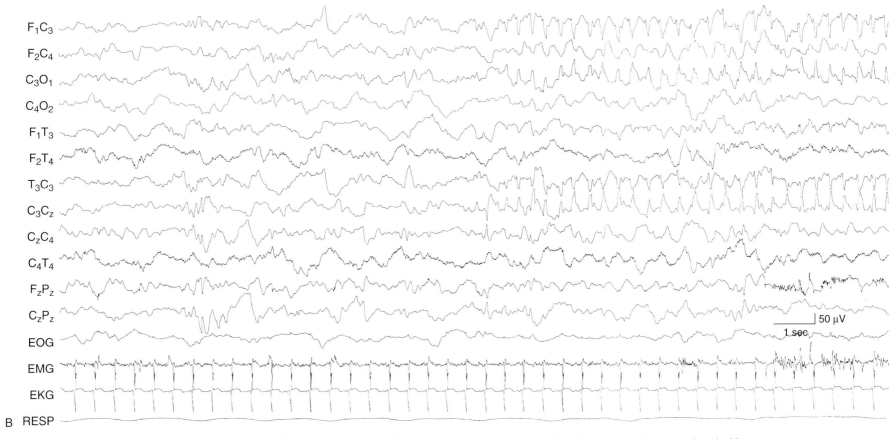

**FIG. 7–1.** *(Continued)* **B:** Later in the recording, an electrical seizure arose from the same region associated with focal clonic activity of the right arm. The background EEG activity is within the range of normal variation. This EEG is from a 41-week CA infant with a left fronto-parietal lobe infarction.

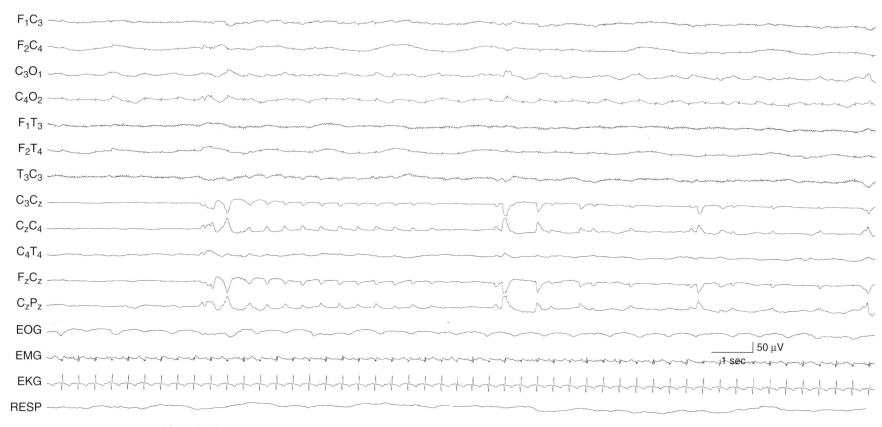

**FIG. 7–2. Discharge duration defines the seizure.** A brief discharge is present in the midline central region with a duration less than 10 seconds. Some sharp waves occur less regularly after the discharge. The background activity is depressed and undifferentiated in this 40-week CA infant with hypoxic–ischemic encephalopathy.

**FIGURES CONTINUE ON THE NEXT PAGE**

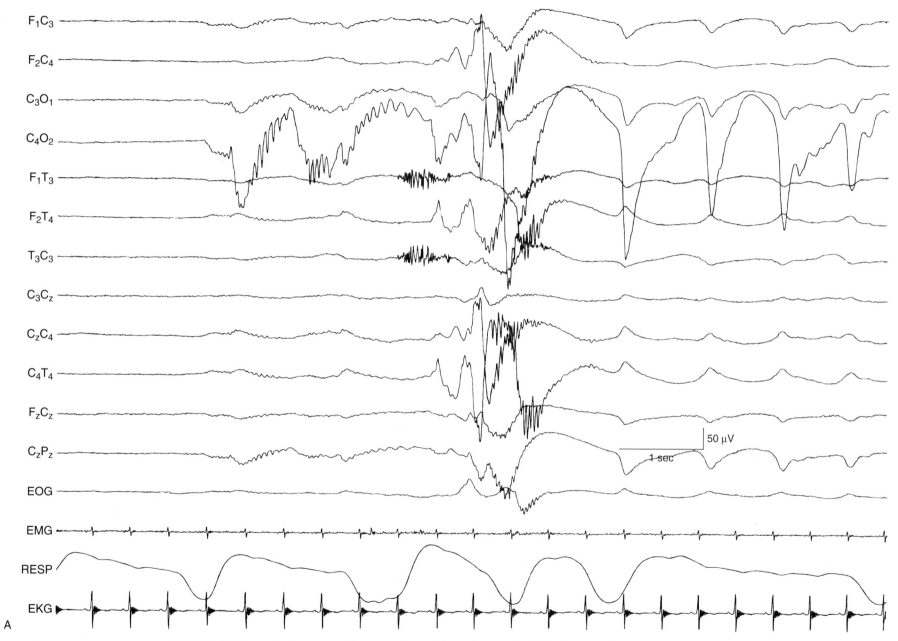

**FIG. 7–3. Seizure discharges in the premature infant.** Segments **A–C** show continuous recordings. **A:** An electrical seizure begins in the right occipital region in this 28-week CA infant.

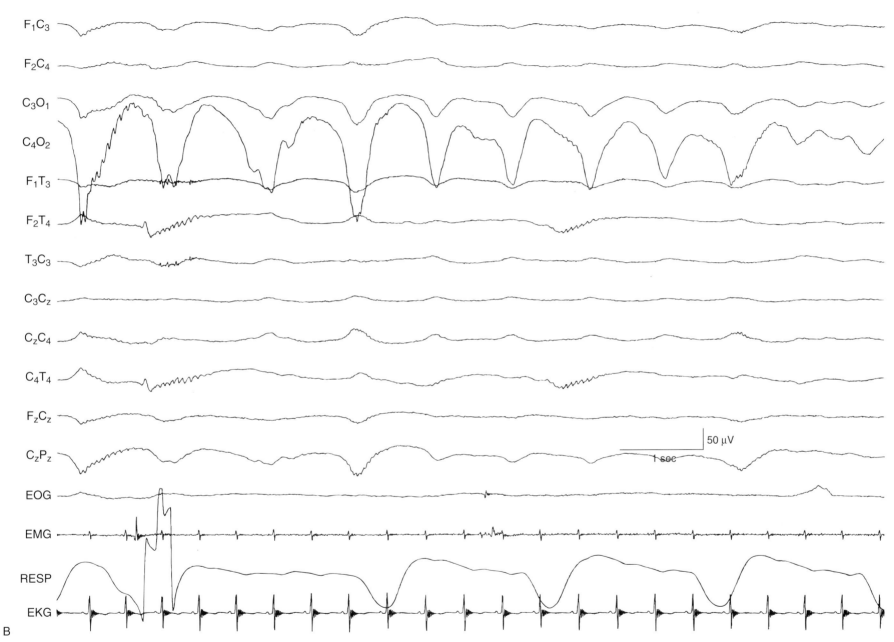

**FIG. 7–3.** *(Continued)* **B:** The discharge persists with gradually reducing amplitude, although the amplitudes are quite high. *(continued)*

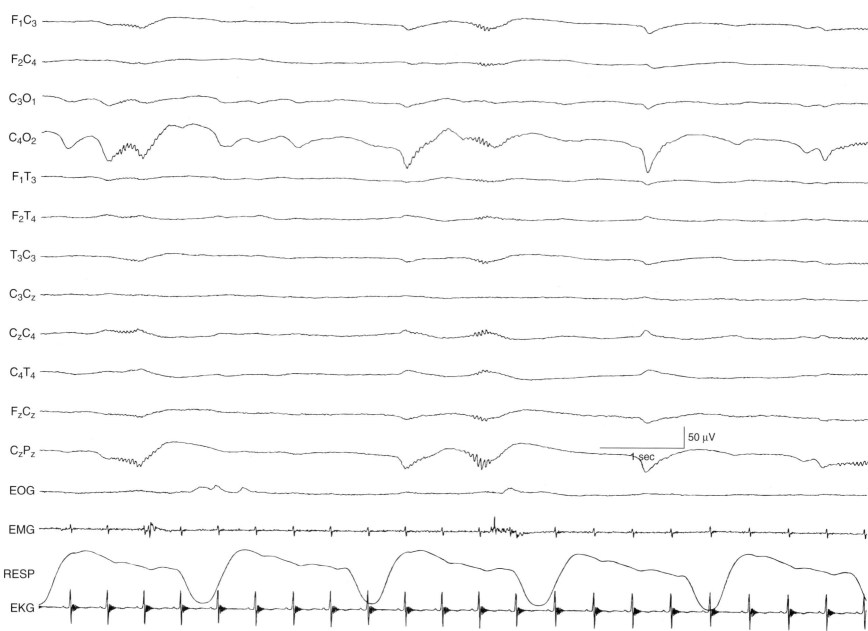

**FIG. 7–3.** *(Continued)* **C:** The seizure discharge subsides.

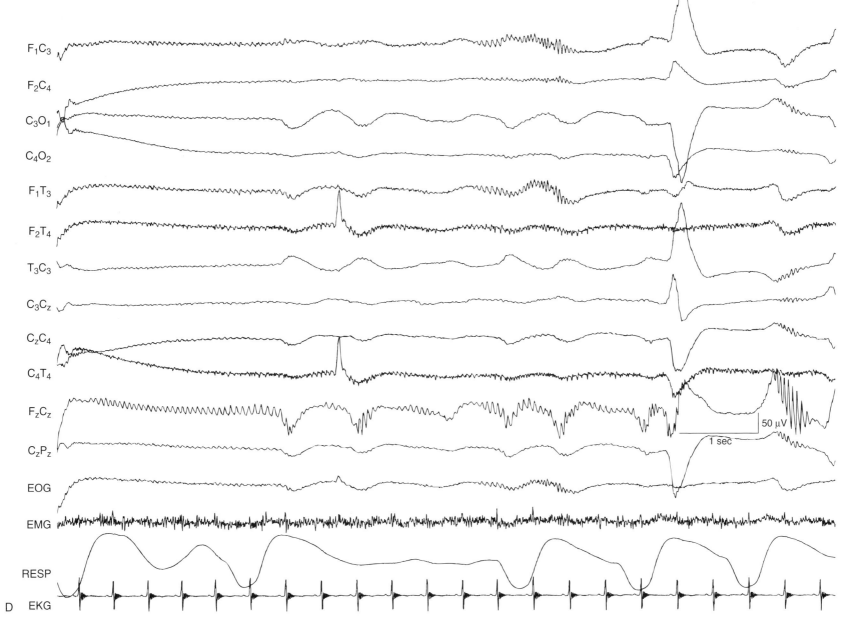

**FIG. 7–3.** *(Continued)* **D:** During the same recording, rhythmic alpha activity occurs in the midline frontal region lateralized to the left. *(continued)*

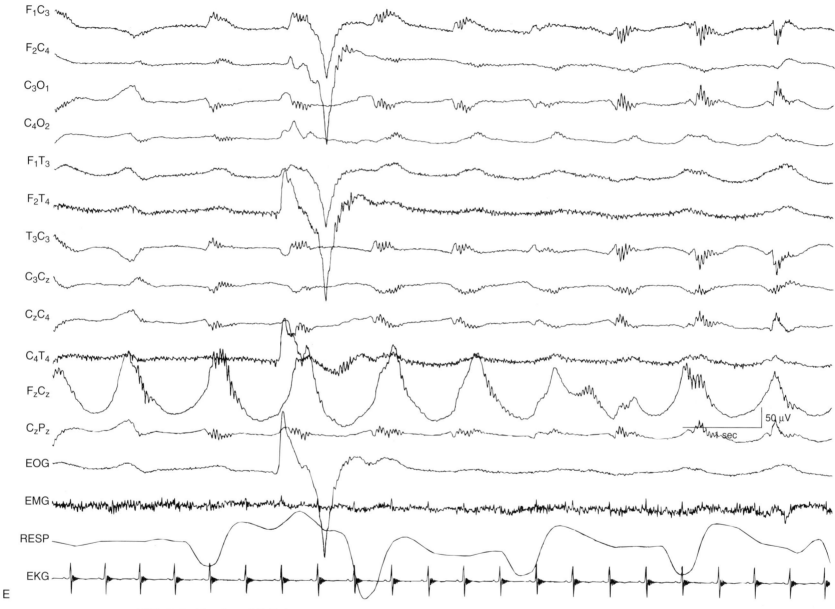

**FIG. 7–3.** *(Continued)* **E:** This segment is continuous with **D** and shows the evolution of the seizure activity to recurrent rhythmic bursts superimposed on very high voltage slow sharp waves. No clinical events occurred with any of the electrical seizure activity.

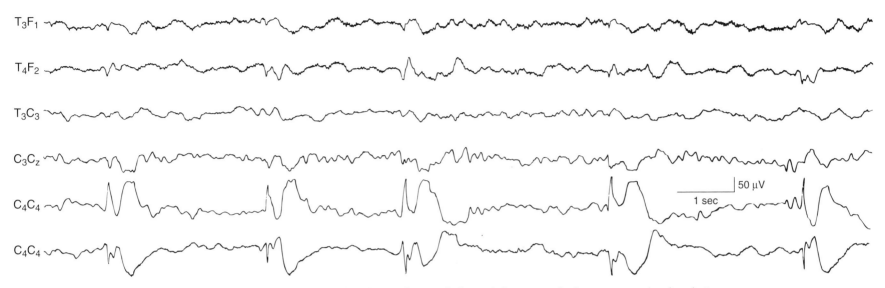

**FIG. 7–4. Seizure discharges with focal myoclonus.** Spike and slow-wave discharges recur at a slow, but regular rate in the right central region. A single, slow, myoclonic flexion of the left arm occurred in close association with each spike and slow-wave discharge. The background activity is within the range of normal variation in this term infant. This is a selected sample from a 12-channel EEG.

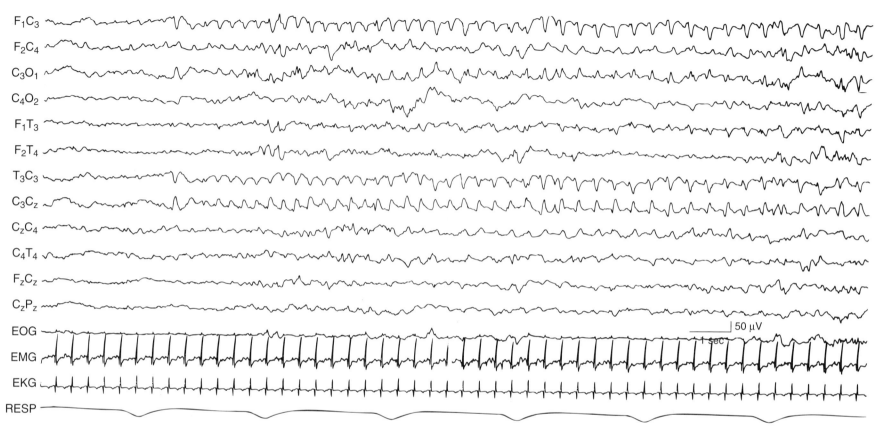

**FIG. 7–5. Central onset of electrical seizure activity.** Rhythmic sharp waves arise in the left central region and remain confined to that region. This electrical activity occurred with a clinical seizure characterized by clonic activity of the right hand in this 40-week CA infant with a left frontal lobe infarction. When the electrical seizure discharge was correlated with computed tomography findings, the site of ictal onset coincided with the periphery of the lesion, a region that perhaps was more capable of generation of such a discharge than the most devitalized cortex at the center of the infarct. The EEG background activity is within the range of normal variation (not shown).

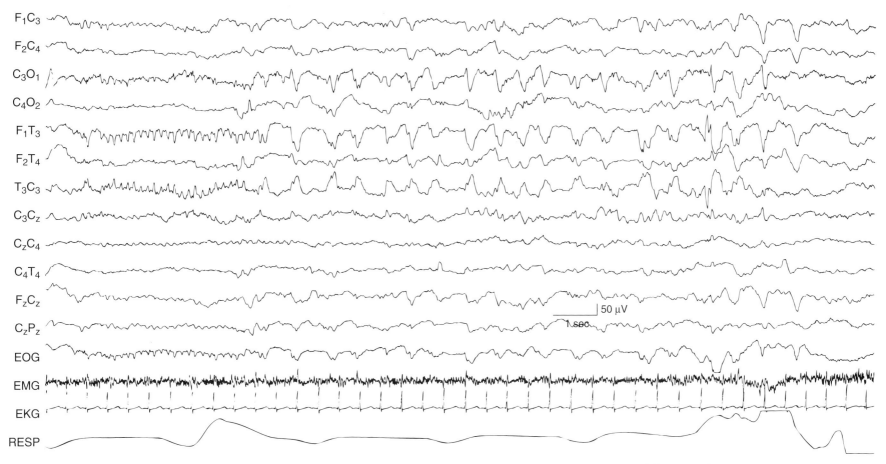

**FIG. 7–6. Temporal onset of electrical seizure activity.** The electrical seizure begins in the left temporal region as low-voltage, fast, rhythmic sharp-wave activity, and then abruptly changes to rhythmic, moderately high voltage, slow activity with sharply contoured waves also involving the posterior region on that side. The seizure is brief, and in the final few seconds of the segments, there is little postictal change. No clinical seizures occurred during this brief electrical event. The interictal EEG background activity is within the range of normal variation (not shown). This sample is from a 40-week CA infant with an intracerebral hemorrhage in the left posterior temporal lobe.

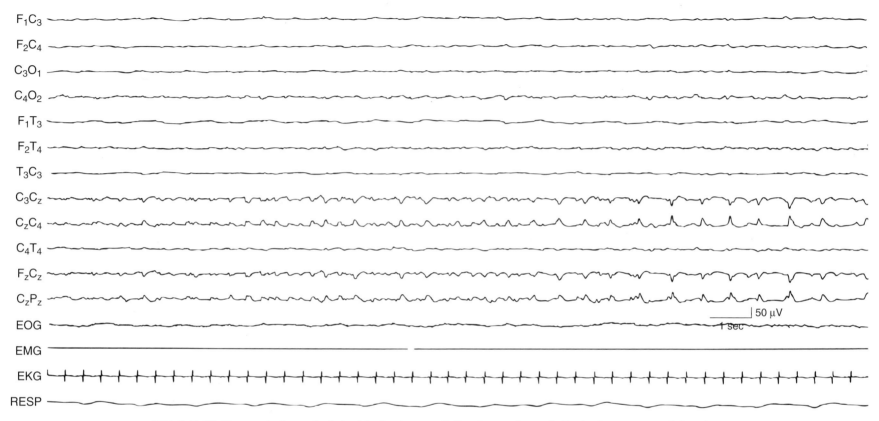

F₁C₃
F₂C₄
C₃O₁
C₄O₂
F₁T₃
F₂T₄
T₃C₃
C₃Cz
CzC₄
C₄T₄
FzCz
CzPz
EOG
EMG
EKG
RESP

50 μV

1 sec

**FIG. 7–7. Midline central onset of electrical seizure activity.** Low-voltage, rhythmic sharp-wave activity arises in the midline central region and remains confined to that region throughout the seizure. Little evidence of this activity appears from electrodes covering adjacent brain regions. The background EEG activity is depressed and undifferentiated. The electrical event can be described as a "seizure discharge of the depressed brain." No clinical seizures occurred in association with the electrical seizure activity. This EEG is from a 38-week CA infant with diffuse cerebral ischemia due to maternal hemorrhage before delivery.

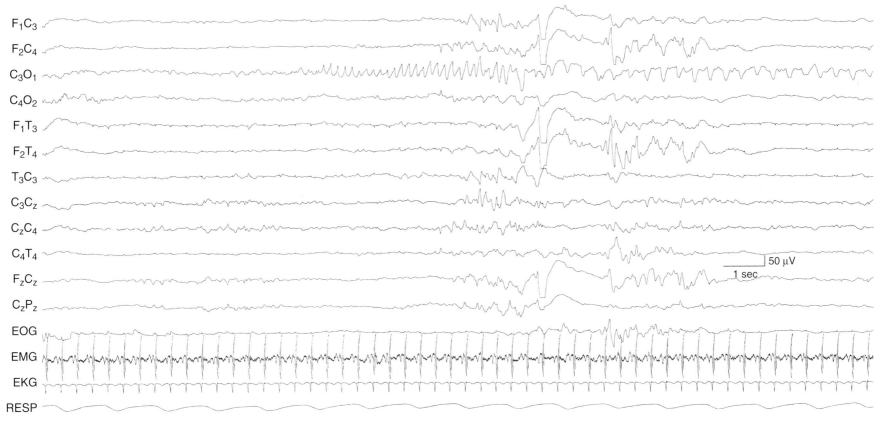

**FIG. 7–8. Occipital onset of electrical seizure activity.** Rhythmic sharp waves arise from the left occipital region with evolution to slower rhythmic waveforms not associated with clinical seizures. The interictal background activity is characterized as a suppression-burst pattern. This EEG is from a 40-week CA infant with meconium aspiration, right hemispheric intracerebral hemorrhage, subarachnoid hemorrhage, and congenital syphilis.

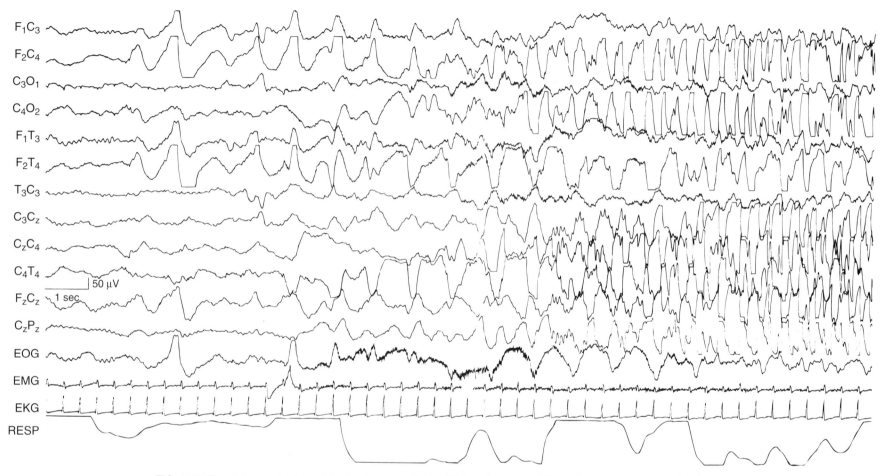

**FIG. 7–9. Frontal onset of electrical seizure activity.** High-voltage, repetitive, slow sharp waves arise in the right frontal region and, after several seconds, appear as faster and sharper discharges that have spread to the right central region. With electrical seizure onset, a clinical seizure begins, characterized by initial extension of the left arm and leg, followed by clonic jerking of the left hand and foot. The interictal EEG background activity is within the range of normal variation (not shown). This occurred in a 40-week CA infant with trisomy 9 and multiple congenital anomalies, including tetralogy of Fallot, absent right kidney, and dysmorphic facial features.

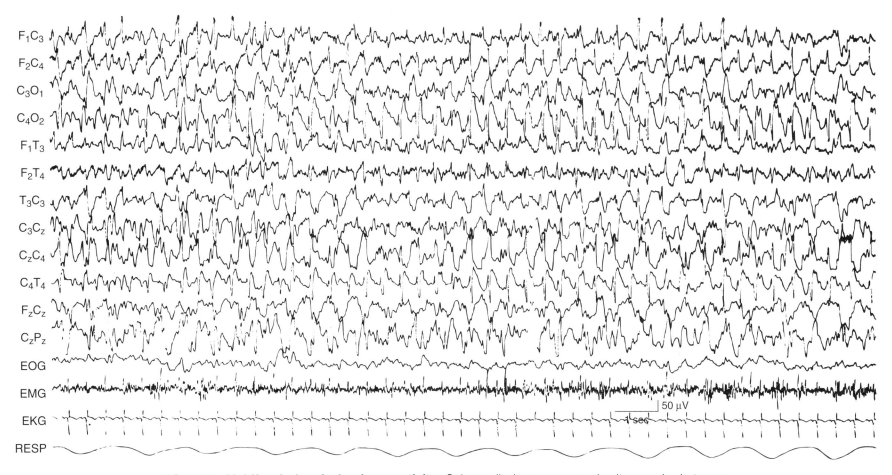

**FIG. 7–10. Multifocal electrical seizure activity.** Seizure discharges occur simultaneously, but asynchronously, in the central regions. No clinical seizures occurred in association with these electrical discharges; the infant had been treated with phenobarbital before EEG recording. The interictal EEG background activity is depressed and undifferentiated (not shown). This EEG is recorded from a 39-week CA infant with hypoglycemia.

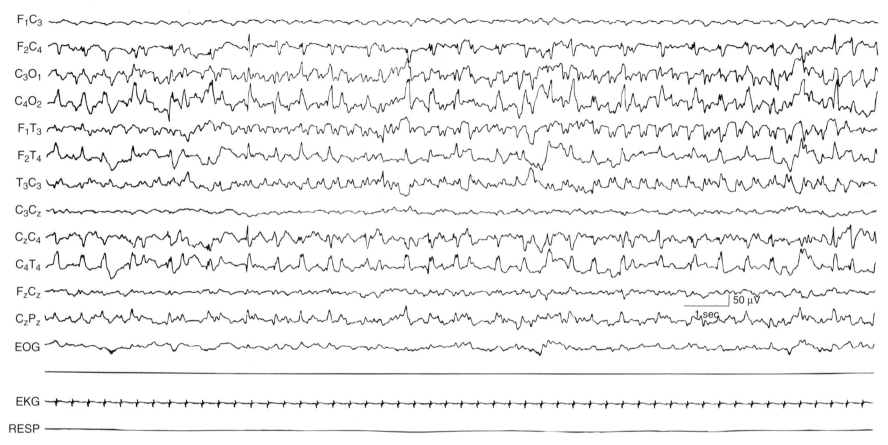

F₁C₃

F₂C₄

C₃O₁

C₄O₂

F₁T₃

F₂T₄

T₃C₃

C₃Cz

CzC₄

C₄T₄

FzCz

CzPz

EOG

EKG

RESP

50 μV

1 sec

**FIG. 7–11. Multifocal electrical seizure activity.** Initially, rhythmic, moderate-voltage, sharp-wave activity arises from the right centrotemporal region. Another seizure discharge arises independently from the left temporal region, characterized by sharp- and slow-wave activity with complex morphology. No clinical seizures occurred with these electrical seizures. The EEG background activity is depressed and undifferentiated (not shown). This EEG is from a 39-week CA infant with meconium aspiration, cardiac failure, and persistent cyanosis and hypoxemia requiring extracorporeal membrane oxygenation.

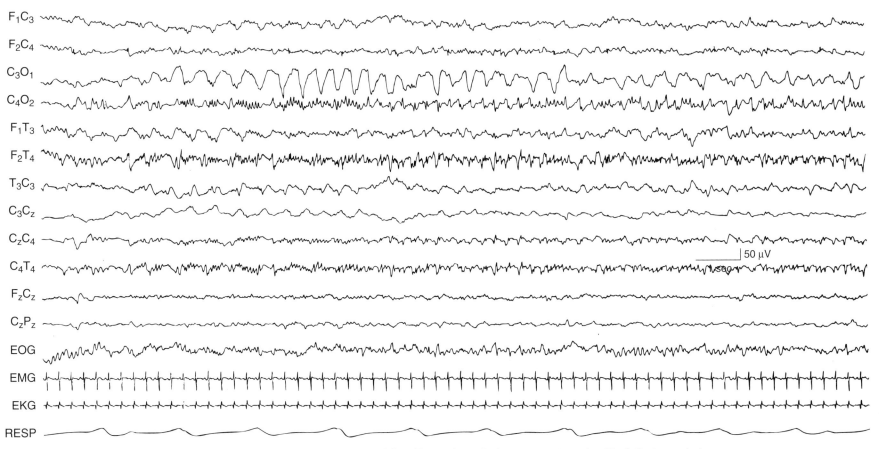

**FIG. 7–12. Multifocal electrical seizure activity.** Two seizure foci are present, each with distinct morphology. Rhythmic, slow, moderate-voltage activity is seen in the left occipital region, and independent, low- to moderate-voltage, rhythmic, fast activity in the right temporo-occipital region. The background activity is depressed and undifferentiated (not shown). No clinical seizures occurred with the electrical seizures. This EEG is from a 4-week-old infant, born at 38 weeks GA (42 weeks CA) with pneumococcal meningitis. Neuroimaging revealed bilateral subdural fluid collections, greater on the right; bilateral parasylvian petechial hemorrhages, and bilateral cerebral edema.

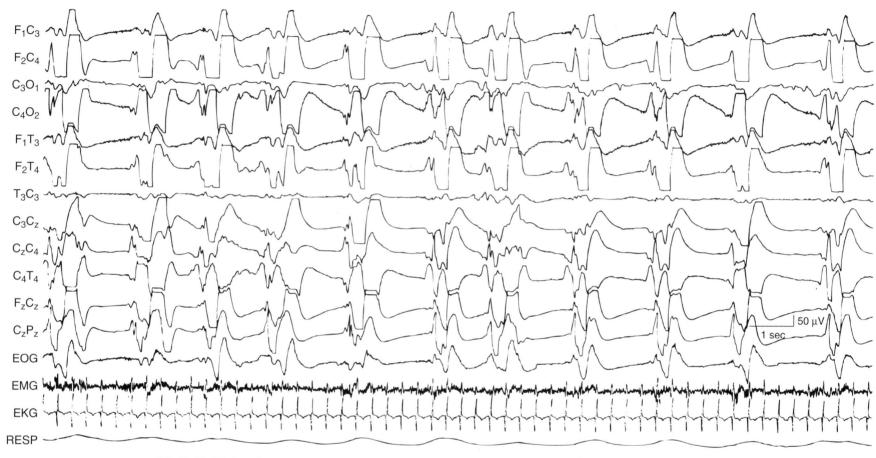

**FIG. 7–13. High-voltage seizure activity.** High-voltage, repetitive, sharp and slow waves, mixed with some spike and slow waves, are present in the right central region with involvement of all of the hemisphere on that side. A clinical seizure coincided with the electrical seizure discharge and was characterized by focal clonic activity of left leg, face, and hand. The background EEG activity was depressed and undifferentiated (not shown). This EEG is from a 40-week CA infant with subarachnoid hemorrhage.

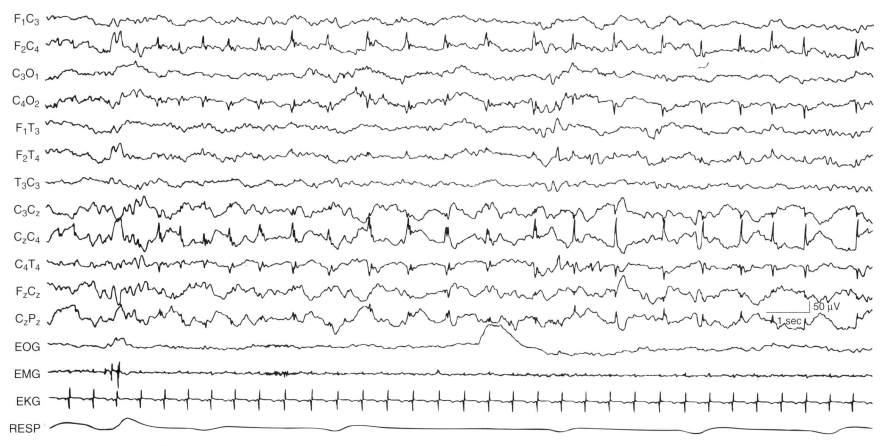

**FIG. 7–14. Spike morphology of seizure discharges.** A seizure discharge arises from the right central region consisting of repetitive spike discharges occurring in association with a clinical seizure characterized by focal clonic activity of the left foot. This EEG is from a 41-week CA infant with group B streptococcal meningitis and associated cerebral infarction of the right posterior temporal and occipital lobes.

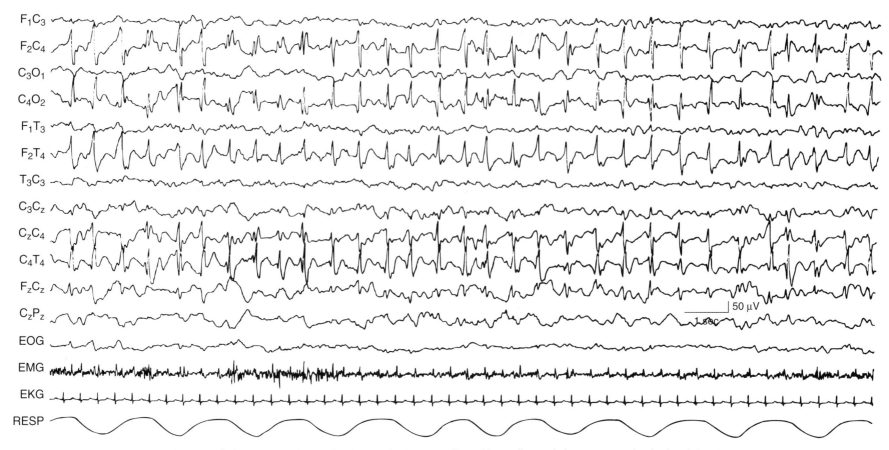

**FIG. 7–15. Spike morphology of seizure discharges.** Repetitive spike and slow waves arise in the right centrotemporal region in association with a clinical seizure characterized by left arm, leg, and face focal clonic activity. The interictal background activity was within the range of normal variation for age (not shown). This EEG is from an 8-week-old, 34-week GA (42-week CA) infant with nonaccidental head trauma resulting in an intracerebral hemorrhage in the right frontal lobe.

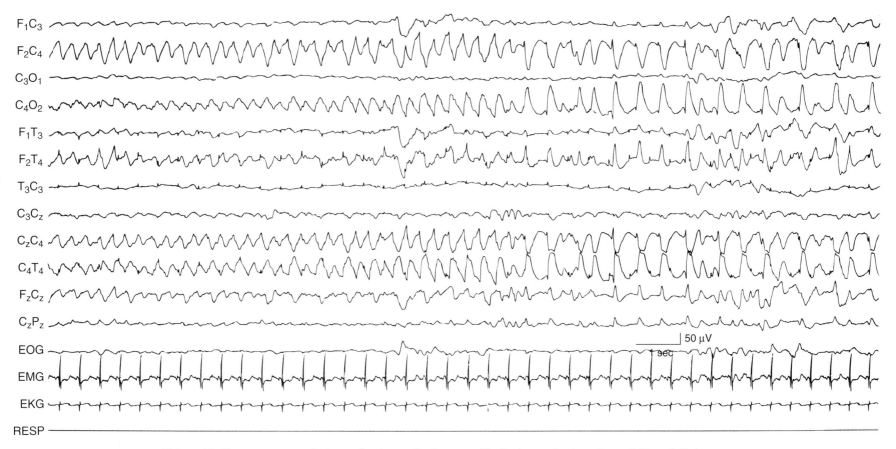

**FIG. 7–16. Slow wave morphology of seizure discharges.** Rhythmic, moderate-voltage, 3-Hz activity is present in the right central region and evolves to seizure activity, which is high in voltage, slower, and mixed with spike discharges. This occurred in association with focal clonic activity of the left hand. The background EEG activity is depressed and undifferentiated. This EEG is from a 38-week CA with meconium aspiration, persistent hypoxemia, and extracorporeal membrane oxygenation support.

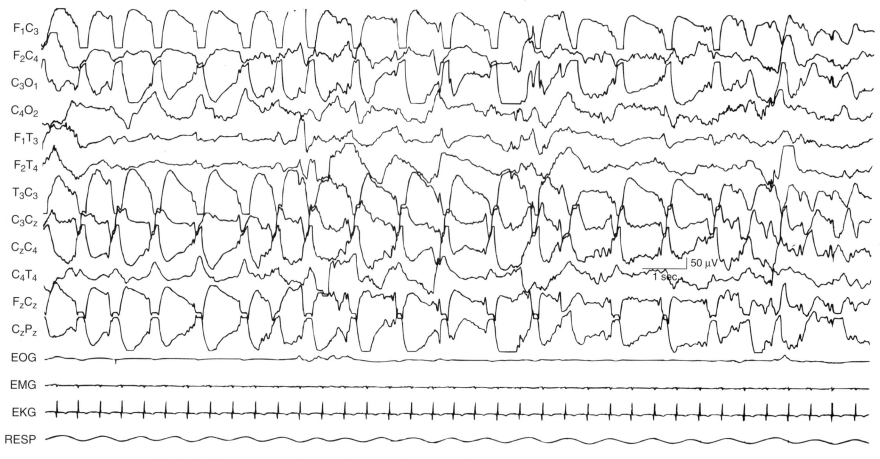

**FIG. 7–17. Slow wave morphology of seizure discharges.** High-voltage, slow rhythmic activity, mixed with occasional spikes, is present in the left central region and occurred in association with the focal clonic activity of the face, arm, and leg on the right. The interictal EEG background activity is within the range of normal variation (not shown). This EEG is from a 42-week CA infant with intraventricular hemorrhage in the left lateral ventricle near the head of the caudate and cerebral edema in the left frontal lobe adjacent to the hemorrhage.

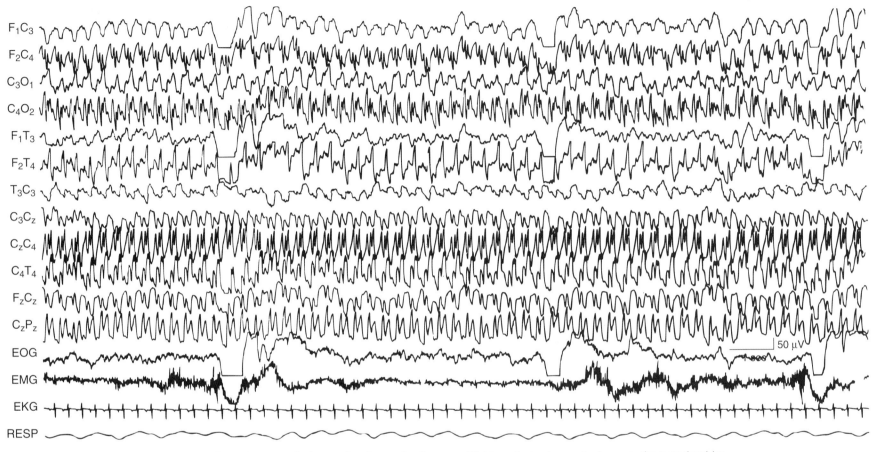

**FIG. 7–18. Complex morphology of seizure discharges.** Right central seizure discharges characterized by rhythmic slow activity with superimposed waves of faster frequency. Independent electrical seizure activity is seen in the right temporal region, consisting of rhythmic sharp waves that do not appear to be reflected in the activity of the central focus. This is associated with a clinical seizure characterized by focal clonic activity of the left arm and leg. The EEG background activity is within the range of normal variation (not shown). The EEG is from a 6-week-old, 37-week GA (43-week CA) infant with a history of congenital renal dysplasia and renal failure. The patient experienced a right frontal lobe infarction with evolution to a porencephalic cyst in that region.

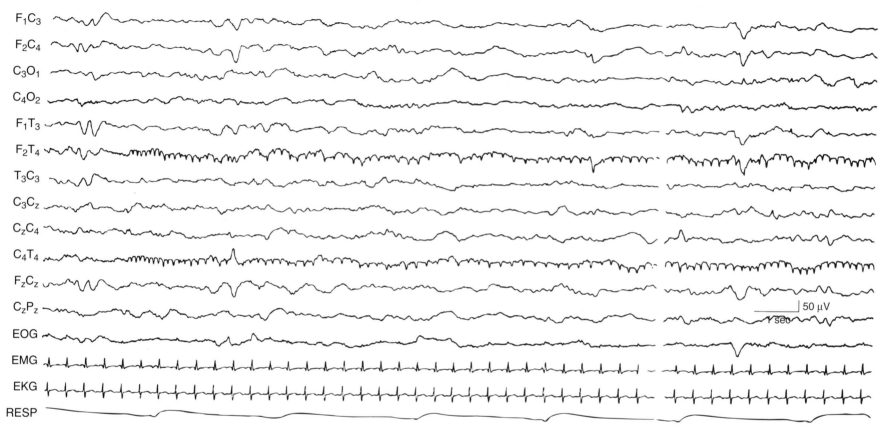

**FIG. 7–19. Highly localized electrical seizures.** Low-voltage, rhythmic, fast spikes arise in the right temporal region and remain confined to that region throughout the seizure. No clinical events were associated with the seizure discharge. The background EEG activity is depressed and undifferentiated. The EEG is from a 40-week CA infant with chronic hypoxemia due to congenital heart disease that included transposition of the great vessels. The patient was treated by balloon atrial septostomy.

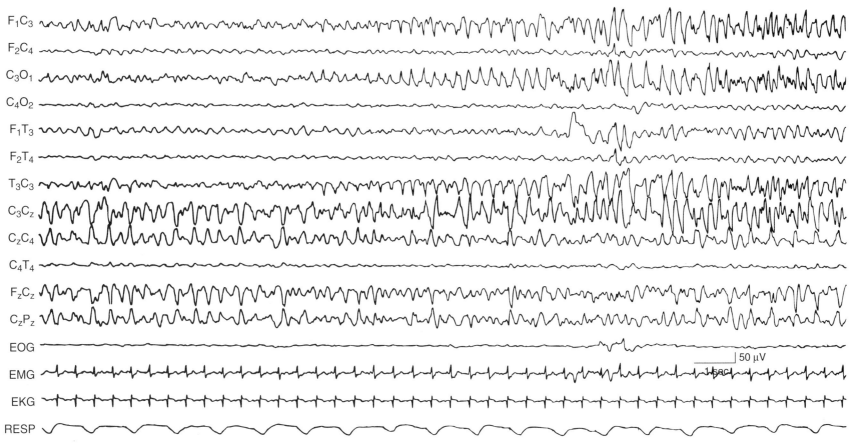

**FIG. 7–20. Spread of electrical seizure activity.** Electrical seizure activity begins in the midline central region (Cz) and then shifts to the left central region (C3), with less involvement at Cz. No clinical seizures were associated with the electrical seizure. The background EEG activity was characterized as suppression-burst (not shown). This EEG is from a 40-week CA infant with hypoxic–ischemic encephalopathy, persistent pulmonary hypertension, hepatic failure, and disseminated intravascular coagulation.

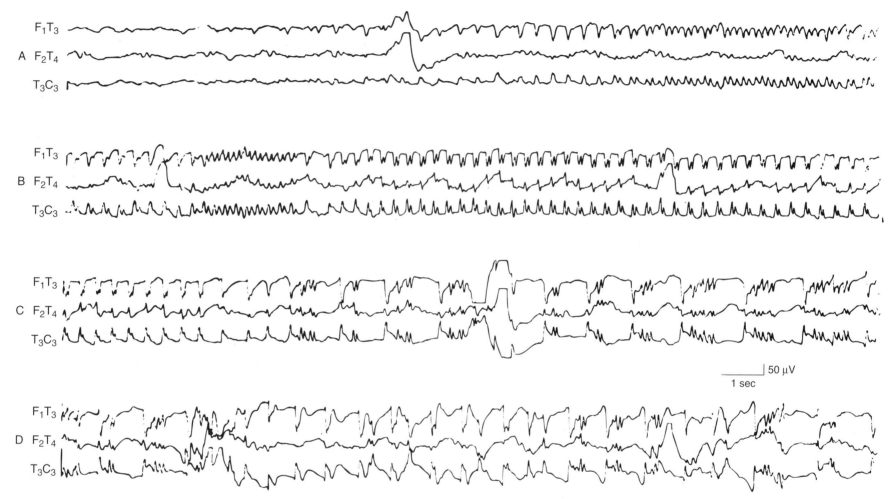

**FIG. 7–21. Evolution in appearance of a single electrical seizure (A–H).** These samples of three selected channels of a 12-channel EEG show a single electrical seizure from beginning to end. The seizure is confined to the left temporal with a changing morphology of the waveforms. No clinical seizures were associated with these electrical seizures. The background activity is depressed and undifferentiated (not shown). This EEG is from a 40-week CA with meconium aspiration, hepatic and liver failure, hypoglycemia, and hypoxic-ischemic encephalopathy.

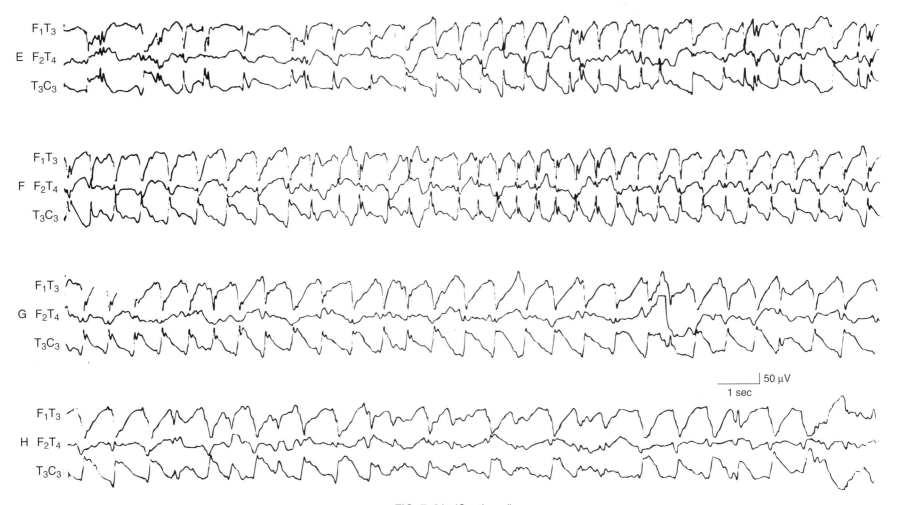

**FIG. 7–21.** (Continued)

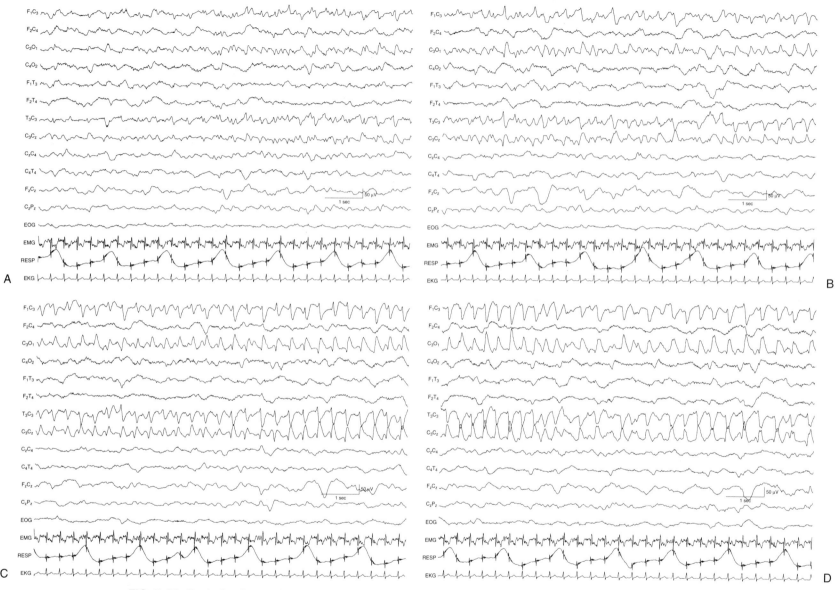

**FIG. 7–22. Evolution in appearance of a single electrical seizure (A–H).** One electrical seizure that lasts approximately 80 sec is shown in eight contiguous samples. The seizure begins as low-voltage rhythmic theta activity in the left central region. A change in frequency and morphology is seen throughout the seizure discharge. The background EEG activity is undifferentiated. This EEG is from a 3-week-old infant, born at 40 weeks GA (43 weeks CA) with pyloric stenosis, intractable vomiting, and multiple electrolyte metabolic disorders.

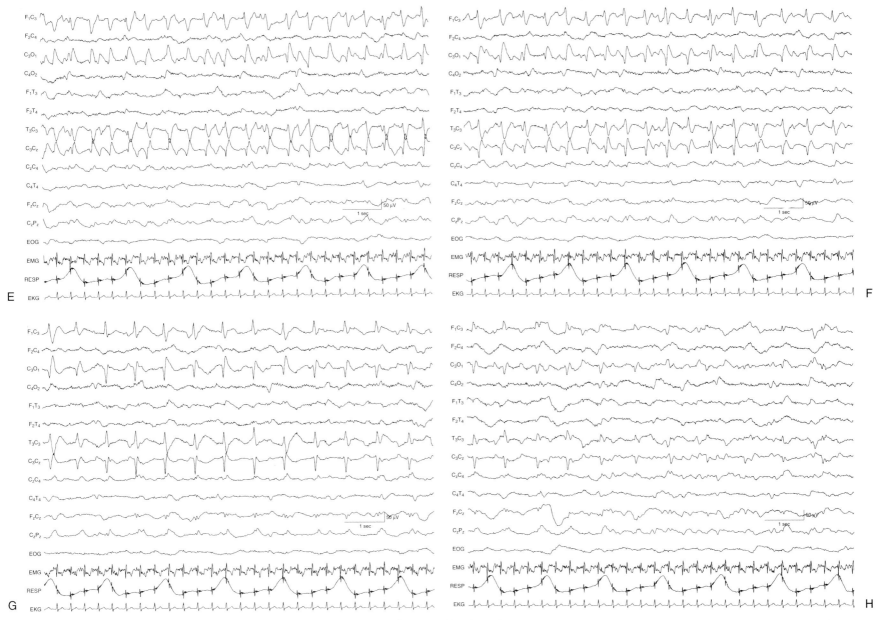

**FIG. 7–22.** *(Continued)*

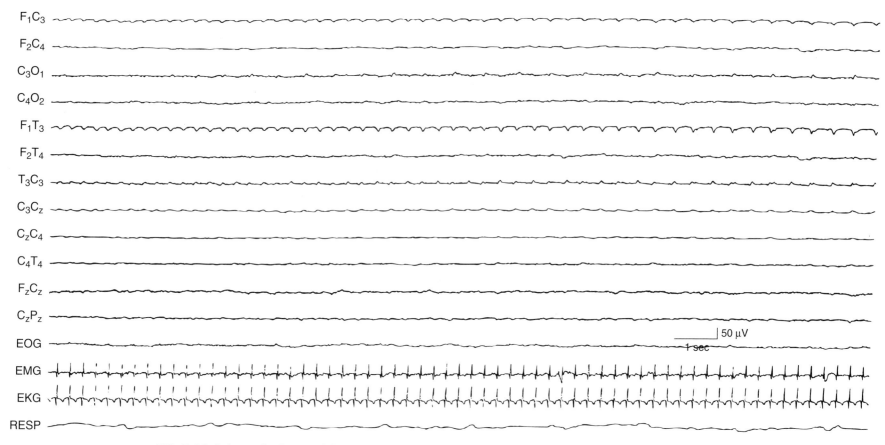

**FIG. 7–23. Seizure discharge of the depressed brain.** Low-voltage, rhythmic, monomorphic, slow sharp waves on the left persist virtually unchanged during the recorded seizure. No clinical seizures occurred during the electrical seizure. The background EEG is depressed and undifferentiated. This EEG is from a 38-week CA infant with persistently low Apgar scores, acidosis, subsequent multisystem organ failure, and hypoxic-ischemic encephalopathy.

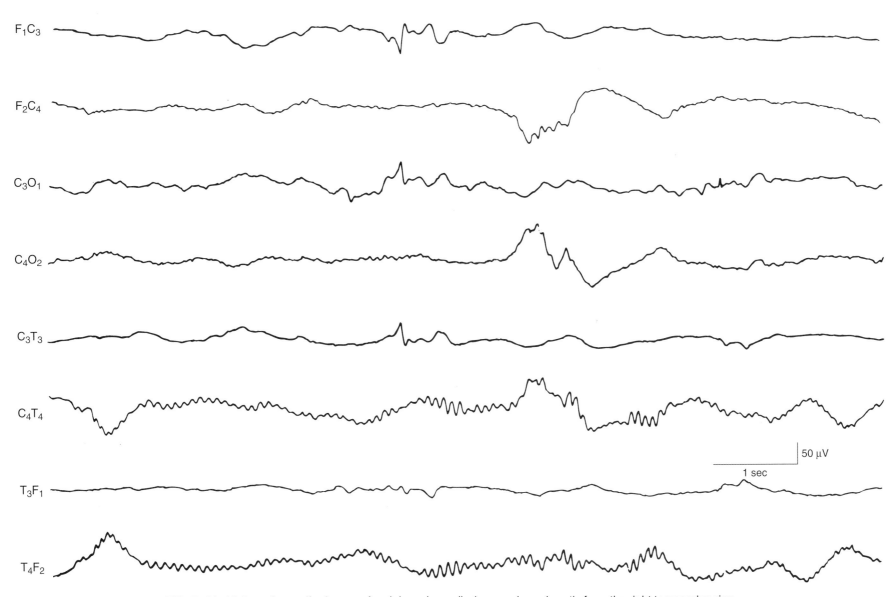

**FIG. 7–24. Alpha seizure discharge.** An alpha seizure discharge arises abruptly from the right temporal region, characterized by rhythmic sinusoidal activity. No clinical seizures were associated with this electrical seizure. The background activity is depressed and undifferentiated. This EEG is from a term infant with hypoxic-ischemic encephalopathy.

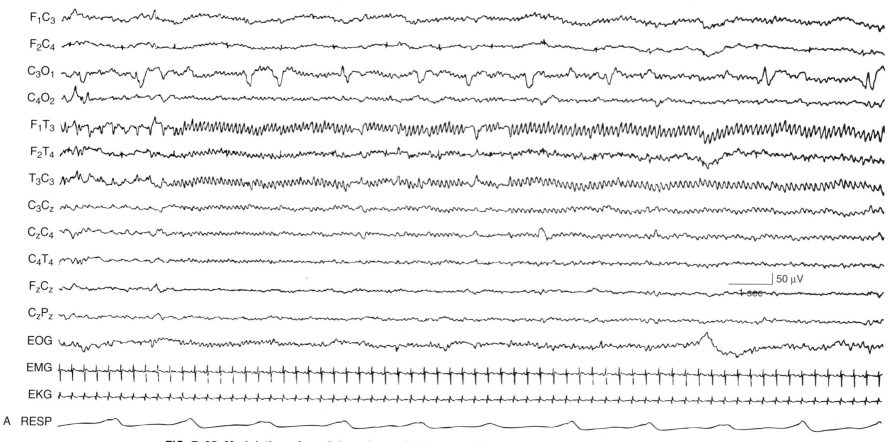

**FIG. 7–25. Modulation of an alpha seizure discharge. A:** A seizure discharge is present in the left temporal region characterized by sinusoidal 10- to 11-Hz rhythmic activity that evolved from rhythmic sharp-wave activity. Independent, semiperiodic slow-wave transients also are present in the left occipital region. No clinical seizures occurred during these electrical seizures. The background activity is depressed and undifferentiated. This EEG is from a 38-week CA with postnatally acquired pneumococcal meningitis.

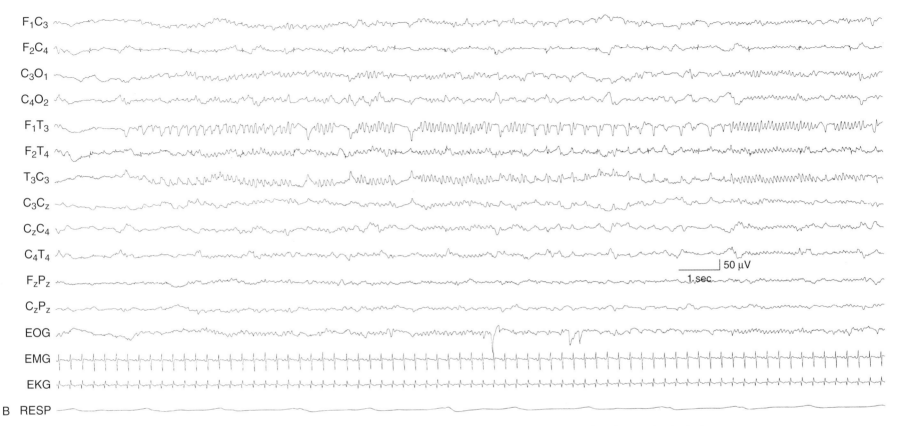

**FIG. 7–25.** *(Continued)* **B:** Later in the same recording the electrical seizure modulated abruptly. As before, no clinical seizures occurred during these electrical seizures.

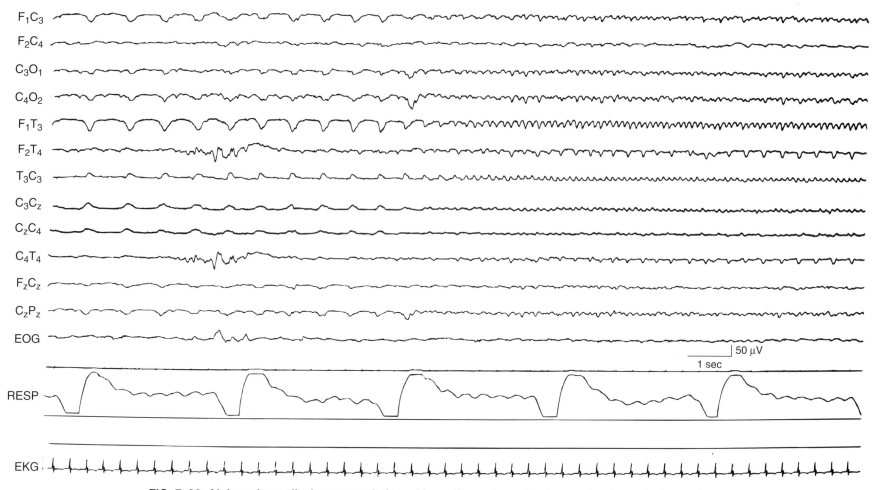

**FIG. 7–26. Alpha seizure discharge coexisting with another seizure discharge.** A seizure discharge characterized by rhythmic 8-Hz sinusoidal activity evolves from rhythmic, slow, sharp-wave activity in the left temporofrontal region. Approximately halfway through this segment of EEG, an independent seizure discharge arises in the right temporal region consisting of low-voltage, rhythmic, slow, monomorphic sharp waves that can be characterized as seizure discharges of the depressed brain. No clinical seizures accompanied these electrical seizures. The background EEG activity is depressed and undifferentiated (not shown). This EEG is from a 12-week-old, former 26-week GA (38-week CA) infant who was initially hospitalized throughout the first 10 weeks of life and then discharged. He was readmitted 2 weeks later with nonaccidental head trauma with computed tomography–demonstrated diffuse and bilateral cerebral edema; focal parenchymal hemorrhages in the left temporal, parietal, and occipital lobes; and posterior fossa subarachnoid hemorrhage.

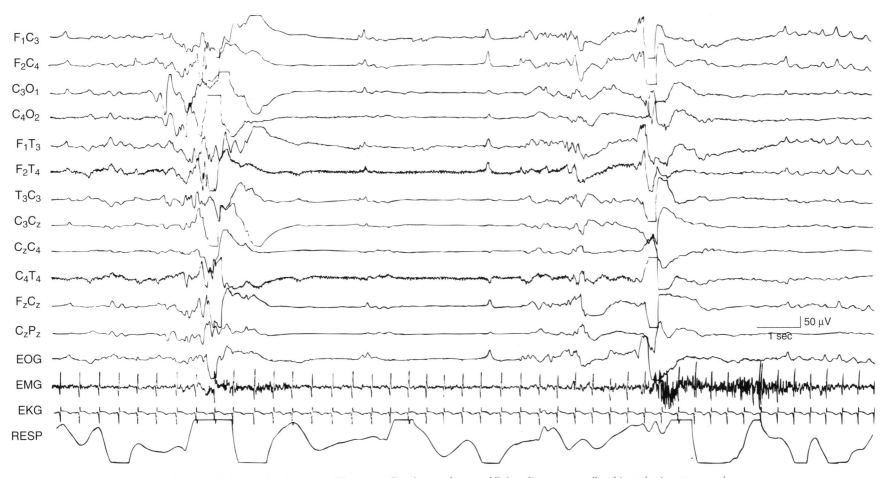

**FIG. 7–27. Seizure discharges with generalized myoclonus.** High voltage generalized transients are associated with myoclonic seizures characterized by brief, axial movements involving the trunk and shoulders. There is increased activity in the electromyogram channel after the occurrence of each generalized transient. Some bursting occurred in the absence of myoclonic movements (not shown). The background activity is characterized by a suppression-burst pattern. This EEG is from a 36-week CA infant with lissencephaly.

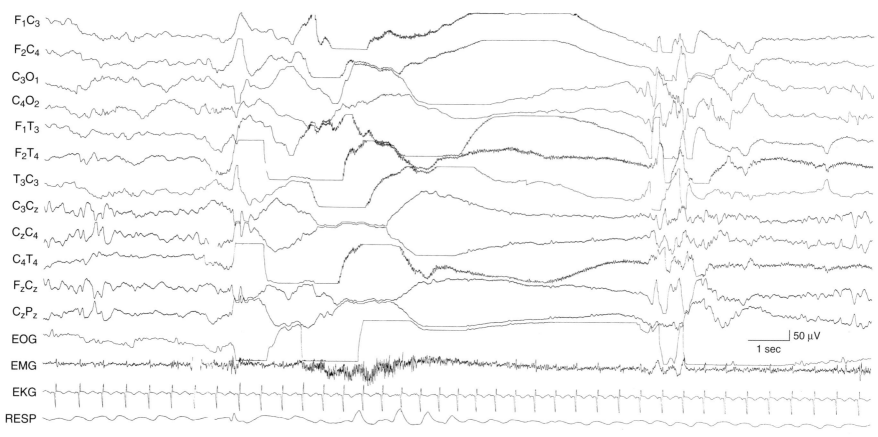

F₁C₃
F₂C₄
C₃O₁
C₄O₂
F₁T₃
F₂T₄
T₃C₃
C₃Cz
CzC₄
C₄T₄
FzCz
CzPz
EOG
EMG
EKG
RESP

50 µV
1 sec

**FIG. 7–28. Generalized voltage attenuation with a spasm.** This infant had a generalized flexor spasm during this brief EEG sample. It was associated with a generalized voltage attenuation. This EEG is from a 39-week CA infant with meconium aspiration, persistent pulmonary hypertension, and hypoxic–ischemic encephalopathy.

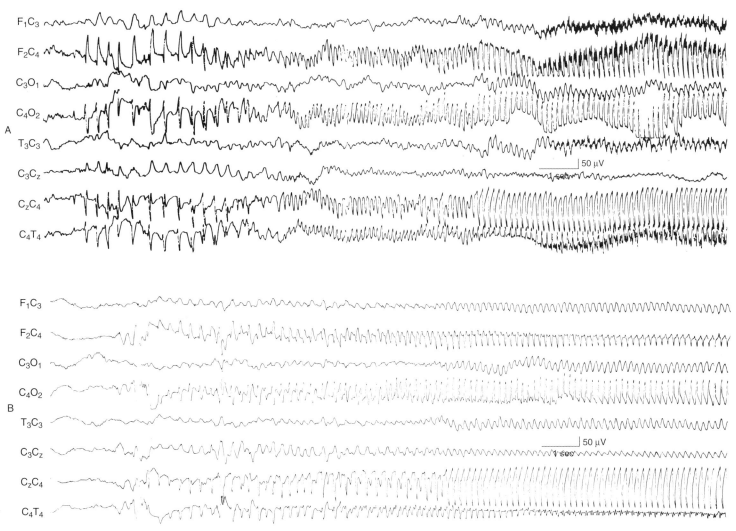

**FIG. 7–29. Response to short-term antiepileptic drug (AED) therapy. A:** Electrical seizure activity arises from the right central region and clinically is associated with a focal clonic seizure of the left arm. This sample of the EEG was recorded before AED therapy. **B:** The infant then received phenobarbital (loading dose, 20 mg/kg, i.v.) and had no further clinical seizures. However, later during continued EEG recording, a recurrence of the electrical seizure activity was seen in the same region as that before AED therapy. No clinical seizures occurred during this electrical seizure. This is considered a "decoupling" of the clinical seizures from the electrical seizures. This EEG is from a 40-week CA infant with a region of focal cortical dysplasia in the right parietal lobe near the midline. (From Hrachovy RA, Mizrahi EM, Kellaway P. Electroencephalography of the newborn. In: Daly DD, Pedley TA, eds. *Current practice of clinical electroencephalography,* 2nd ed. New York: Raven Press, 1990:201–241, with permission.)

# Bibliography

Aicardi J. Early myoclonic encephalopathy. In: Roger S, Dravet C, Bureau M, et al., eds. *Epileptic syndromes in infancy, childhood, and adolescence.* London: John Libbey, 1985:12–22.

Aicardi J. Early myoclonic encephalopathy (neonatal myoclonic encephalopathy). In: Roger J, Bureau M, Dravet C, et al., eds. *Epileptic syndromes in infancy, childhood, and adolescence,* 2nd ed. London: John Libbey, 1992:13–23.

Aicardi J, Ohtahara S. Severe nconatal epilepsies with suppression-burst pattern. In: Roger J, Bureau M, Dravet C, et al., eds. *Epileptic syndromes in infancy, childhood, and adolescence,* 3rd ed. London: John Libbey, 2002:33–44.

Albala BJ, Moshe SL, Okada, R. Kainic-acid-induced seizures: a developmental study. *Brain Res* 1984;315:139–148.

American Clinical Neurophysiology Society. Minimum technical standards for pediatric electroencephalography. *J Clin Neurophysiol* 1986;3:139–143.

Anderson CM, Torres F, Faoro A. The EEG of the premature. *Electroencephalogr Clin Neurophysiol* 1985;60:95–105.

Biagioni E, Ferrari F, Boldrini A, et al. Electroclinical correlation in neonatal seizures. *Eur J Paediatr Neurol* 1998;2:117–125.

Blume WT, Dreyfus-Brisac C. Positive rolandic sharp waves in neonatal EEG: Types and significance. *Electroencephalogr Clin Neurophysiol* 1982;53:277–282.

Boylan GB, Pressler RM, Rennie J, et al. Outcome of electroclinical, electrographic, and clinical seizures in the newborn infant. *Dev Med Child Neurol* 1999;41:819–825.

Boylan GB, Rennie JM, Pressler RM, et al. Phenobarbitone, neonatal seizures, and video-EEG. *Arch Dis Child Fetal Neonatal Ed* 2002;86:F165–F170.

Brittenham DM. Artifacts. In: Daly DD, Pedley TA, eds. *Current practice of clinical electroencephalography.* 2nd edition. New York: Raven Press, 1990:85–105.

Burke JB. Prognostic significance of neonatal convulsions. *Arch Dis Child* 1954;29:342–345.

Bye AM, Cunningham CA, Chee K, et al. Outcome of neonates with electrographically identified seizures, or at risk of seizures. *Pediatr Neurol* 1997;16:225–231.

Bye AM, Flanagan D. Spatial and temporal characteristics of neonatal seizures. *Epilepsia* 1995;36:1009–1016.

Cadilhac J, Passouant P, Ribstein M. Convulsions in the newborn: EEG and clinical aspects. *Electroencephalogr Clin Neurophysiol* 1959;11:604.

Challamel M-J, Isnard H, Brunon AM, et al. Asymetrie EEG transitoire a l'entrée dans le sommeil calme chez le nouveau-né: Étude sur 75 observations. *Rev Electroencephalogr Neurophysiol Clin* 1984;14:17–23.

Chequer RS, Tharp BR, Dreimane D, et al. Prognostic value of EEG in neonatal meningitis: Retrospective study of 29 infants. *Pediatr Neurol* 1992;8:417–422.

Cilio MR, Sogawa Y, Cha BH, et al. Long-term effects of status epilepticus in the immature brain are specific for age and model. *Epilepsia* 2003;44:518–528.

Clancy RR. The contribution of EEG to the understanding of neonatal seizures. *Epilepsia* 1996;suppl 1:S52–S59.

Clancy RR, Bergqvist AGC, Dlugos DJ. Neonatal electroencephalography. In: Ebersole JS, Pedley TA. *Current practice of clinical electroencephalography,* 3rd edition. Philadelphia: Lippincott Williams & Wilkins, 2003:160–245.

Clancy RR, Chung HJ, Temple JP. Neonatal electroencephalography. In: Sperling MR, Clancy RR, eds. *Atlas of electroencephalography.* New York: Elsevier, 1993:182.

Clancy RR, Legido A. The exact ictal and interictal duration of electroencephalographic neonatal seizures. *Epilepsia* 1987;28:537–541.

Clancy RR, Legido A, Lewis D. Occult neonatal seizures. *Epilepsia* 1988;29:256–261.

Clancy RR, Tharp BR. Positive rolandic sharp waves in the electroencephalograms of premature neonates with intraventricular hemorrhage. *Electroencephalogr Clin Neurophysiol* 1984;57:395–404.

Commission on Classification and Terminology of the International League against Epilepsy. Proposal for revised classificaion of epilepsies and epileptic syndromes. *Epilepsia* 1989;30:389–399.

Connell JA, Oozeer R, Dubowitz V. Continuous 4-channel EEG monitoring: a guide to interpretation, with normal values, in preterm infants. *Neuropediatrics* 1978;8:138–145.

Cukier F, Andre M, Monod N, et al. Apport de l'EEG au diagnostic des hemorragies intra-ventriculaires du prématuré. *Rev Electroencephalogr Neurophysiol Clin* 1972;2:318–322.

da Costa J, Lombroso CT. Neurophysiological correlates of neonatal intracranial hemorrhage. *Electroencephalogr Clin Neurophysiol* 1980;50:183–184.

de Rogalski Landrot I, Minokoshi M, Silveira DC, et al. Recurrent neonatal seizures: relationship of pathology to the electroencephalogram and cognition. *Brain Res Dev Brain Res* 2001;129:27–38.

De Weerd AW, Despand PA, Plouin P. Neonatal EEG: Recommendations for the practice of clinical neurophysiology: Guidelines of the International Federation of Clinical Neurophysiology. *Electroencephalogr Clin Neurophysiol* 1999;suppl 52:149–157.

Dehan M, Quilleron D, Navelet Y, et al. Les convulsions du cinquième jour de vie: un nouveau syndrome? *Arch Fr Pediatr* 1977;34:730–742.

DeMyer W, White PT. EEG in holoprosencephaly (arhinencephaly). *Arch Neurol* 1964;11:507–520.

DeMyer W, Zeman W. Alobar holoprosencephaly (arhinencephaly) with median cleft lip and palate: Clinical, electroencephalographic and nosologic considerations. *Confin Neurol* 1963;23:1–36.

Douglass LM, Wu JY, Rosman NP, et al. Burst suppression electroencephalogram pattern in the newborn: Predicting the outcome. *J Child Neurol* 2002;17:403–408.

Dreyfus-Brisac C. Activité électrique cérébrale du foetus et du tres jeune prématuré: IV Congr. Int. Electroencephalogr. Neurophysiol. Clin. *Acta Med Belg Ed* 1957:163–171.

Dreyfus-Brisac C. Electroencephalography in infants. In: Linneweh F, ed. *Die physiologische Entwicklung des Kindes*. Berlin: Springer, 1959:29–40.

Dreyfus-Brisac C. The electroencephalogram of the premature infant. *World Neurol* 1962;3:5–15.

Dreyfus-Brisac C. The electroencephalogram of the premature infant and full-term newborn: Normal and abnormal development of waking and sleeping patterns. In: Kellaway P, Peters I, eds. *Neurological and electroencephalographic correlative studies in infancy*. New York: Grune & Stratton, 1964:186–206.

Dreyfus-Brisac C. Sleep ontogenesis in early human prematurity from 24 to 27 weeks of conceptional age. *Dev Psychobiol* 1968;1:162–169.

Dreyfus-Brisac C. Ontogenesis of sleep in human prematures after 32 weeks of conceptional age. *Dev Psychobiol* 1970;3:91–121.

Dreyfus-Brisac C. Ontogenesis of brain bioelectrical activity and sleep organization in neonates and infants. In: Faulkner F, Tanner JM, eds. *Human growth. Vol. 3: Neurobiology and nutrition*. New York: Plenum Press, 1978:157–182.

Dreyfus-Brisac C, Blanc C. Électroencéphalogramme et maturation cerebrale. *Encephale* 1956;45:205–241.

Dreyfus-Brisac C, Fischgold H, Samson-Dollfus D, et al. Veille, sommeil, réactivité sensorielle chez le prématuré, le nouveau-né et le nourrisson. *Electroencephalogr Clin Neurophysiol Suppl* 1957;6:417–440.

Dreyfus-Brisac C, Flescher J, Plassart E. L'électroencéphalogramme: Critère d' âge conceptionnel du nouveau-né à terme et du prématuré. *Biol Neonat* 1962;4:154–173.

Dreyfus-Brisac C, Monod N. Electroclinical studies of status epilepticus and convulsions in the newborn. In Kellaway P, Petersen I, eds: *Neurological and electroencephalographic correlative studies in infancy*. New York: Grune & Stratton, 1964:250–272.

Dreyfus-Brisac C, Monod N. Sleeping behavior in abnormal newborn infants. *Neuropädiatrie* 1970;1:354–366.

Dreyfus-Brisac C, Monod N, Salama P, et al. L'EEG dans les six premiers mois de la vie, aprés réanimation prolongée et état de mal néonatal: Recherches d'éléments de prognostic: Vth International Congress on Electroencephalography and Clinical Neurophysiology, Rome. *Excerpta Med Int Congr Ser* 1961;37:228–229.

Ellingson RJ. Electroencephalograms of normal full-term newborns immediately after birth with observations on arousal and visual evoked responses. *Electroencephalogr Clin Neurophysiol* 1958;10:31–50.

Ellingson RJ. EEGs of premature and full-term newborns. In: Klass DW, Daly DD, eds. *Current practice of clinical electroencephalography*. New York: Raven Press, 1979:149–177.

Engel R. *Abnormal electroencephalograms in the neonatal period*. Springfield, Ill.: Charles C Thomas, 1978.

Engel R, Butler BV. Appraisal of conceptual age of newborn infants by electroencephalographic methods. *J Pediatr* 1963;63:386–393.

Fenichel GM, Olson BJ, Fitzpatrick JE. Heart rate changes in convulsive and nonconvulsive apnea. *Ann Neurol* 1979;7:577–582.

Frost JD. Triaxial vector accelerometry: a method for quantifying tremor and ataxia. *IEEE Trans Biomed Eng* 1978;25:17–27.

Gibbs FA, Gibbs EL. *Atlas of electroencephalography. Vol 2: Epilepsy*. Cambridge, Mass.: Addison-Wesley, 1952.

Glauser TA, Clancy RR. Adequacy of routine EEG examinations in neonates with clinically suspected seizures. *J Child Neurol* 1992;7:215–220.

Graziani LJ, Streletz LJ, Baumgart S, et al. Predictive value of neonatal electroencephalograms before and during extracorporeal membrane oxygenation. *J Pediatr* 1994;125:969–975.

Hagne I. Development of the EEG in normal infants during the first year of life. *Acta Paediatr Scand Suppl* 1972;232:1–53.

Hahn JS, Monyer H, Tharp BR. Interburst interval measurements in the EEGs of premature infants with normal neurological outcome. *Electroencephalogr Clin Neurophysiol* 1989;73:410–418.

Hanley J. A step-by-step approach to neonatal EEG. *Am J EEG Technol* 1981;121:1–13.

Harris R, Tizard JPM. The electroencephalogram in neonatal convulsions. *J Pediatr* 1960;57:502–520.

Hayakawa F, Watanabe K, Hakamada S, et al. FZ theta/alpha bursts: A transient EEG pattern in healthy newborns. *Electroencephalogr Clin Neurophysiol* 1987;67:27–31.

Holmes GL. Seizure-induced neuronal injury: animal data. *Neurology* 2002;9(suppl 5):S3–S6.

Holmes GL, Ben-Ari Y. The neurobiology and consequences of epilepsy in the developing brain. *Pediatr Res* 2002;49:320–325.

Holmes GL, Khazipov R, Ben-Ari Y. Seizure-induced damage in the developing human: relevance of experimental models. *Prog Brain Res* 2002;135:321–334.

Holmes GL, Lombroso CT. Prognostic value of background patterns in the neonatal EEG. *J Clin Neurophysiol* 1993;10:323–352.

Holmes G, Rowe J, Hafford J, et al. Prognostic value of the electroencephalogram in neonatal asphyxia. *Electroencephalogr Clin Neurophysiol* 1982;53:60–72.

Hrachovy RA. Development of the normal electroencephalogram. In: Levin KH, Luders HO, eds. *Comprehensive clinical neurophysiology*. Philadelphia: WB Saunders, 2000:387–413.

Hrachovy RA, Frost JD, Jr, Kellaway P. Hypsarrhythmia: variations on the theme. *Epilepsia* 1984;25:317–325.

Hrachovy RA, Mizrahi EM, Kellaway P. Electroencephalography of the newborn. In: Daly DD, Pedley TA, eds. *Current practice of clinical electroencephalography*. 2nd edition. New York: Raven Press, 1990:201–241.

Hrachovy RA, O'Donnell D. The significance of excessive rhythmic alpha and/or theta frequency activity in the EEG of the neonate. *Clin Neurophysiol* 1999;110:438–444.

Hughes JR Jr, Fino JJ, Hart LA. Premature temporal theta (PT2). *Electroencephalogr Clin Neurophysiol* 1987;67:7–15.

Jasper HH. The ten-twenty electrode system of the International Federation. *Electroencephalogr Clin Neurophysiol* 1958;10:371–373.

Kagawa N. EEG recording in the neonate. *Am J EEG Technol* 1973;13:163–176.

Kellaway P. Orderly approach to visual analysis: Elements of the normal EEG and their characteristics in children and adults. In: Ebersole JS, Pedley TA, eds. *Current practice of clinical electroencephalography*. 3rd edition. Philadelphia: Lippincott Williams & Wilkins, 2003:100–159.

Kellaway P, Crawley JW. *A primer of electroencephalography of infants, sections I & II: Methodology and criteria of normality*. Houston, TX: Baylor University College of Medicine, 1964.

Kellaway P, Hrachovy RA. Electroencephalography. In: Swaiman KF, Wright FS, eds. *The practice of pediatric neurology*. 2nd edition. St. Louis, Mo.: Mosby, 1982:96–114.

Klinger G, Chin CN, Otsubo H, et al. Prognostic value of EEG in neonatal bacterial meningitis. *Pediatr Neurol* 2001;24:28–31.

Knauss TA, Carlson CB. Neonatal paroxysmal monorhythmic alpha activity. *Arch Neurol* 1978;35:104–107.

Kumar P, Gupta R, Shankaran S, et al. EEG abnormalities in survivors of neonatal ECMO: Its role as a predictor of neurodevelopmental outcome. *Am J Perinatol* 1999;16:245–250.

Laroia N, Guillet R, Burchfield J, et al. EEG background as predictor of electrographic seizures in high-risk neonates. *Epilepsia* 1998;39:545–551.

Levy SR, Berg AT, Testa FM, et al. Comparison of digital and conventional EEG interpretation. *J Clin Neurophysiol* 1998;15:476–480.

Lombroso CT. Quantified electrographic scales on 10 pre-term healthy newborns followed up to 40–43 weeks of conceptional age by serial polygraphic recordings. *Electroencephalogr Clin Neurophysiol* 1979;46:460–474.

Lombroso CT. Neonatal electroencephalography. In: Niedermeyer E, Lopez da Silva F, eds. *Electroencephalography: Basic principles, clinical applications and related fields.* Baltimore: Urban & Schwarzenberg, 1982:599–637.

Lombroso CT. Neonatal polygraphy in full-term and premature infants: A review of normal and abnormal findings. *J Clin Neurophysiol* 1985;2:105–155.

Lombroso CT. Neonatal seizures: a clinician's overview. *Brain Dev* 1996a;18:1–28.

Lombroso CT. Neonatal seizures: historic note and present controversies. *Epilepsia* 1996b;suppl 3:5–13.

Maheshwari MC, Jeavons PM. The prognostic implications of suppression-burst activity in the EEG in infancy. *Epilepsia* 1975;16:127–131.

Marret S, Parain D, Samson-Dollfus D, et al. Positive rolandic sharp waves and periventricular leukomalacia in the newborn. *Neuropediatrics* 1986;17:199–202.

McBride MC, Laroia N, Guillet R. Electrographic seizures in neonates correlate with poor neurodevelopmental outcome. *Neurology* 2000;55:506—513.

Mikati MA, Feraru E, Krishnamoorthy K, et al. Neonatal herpes simplex meningoencephalitis: EEG investigations and clinical correlates. *Neurology* 1990;40:1433–1437.

Mizrahi EM. Neonatal electroencephalography: Clinical features of the newborn, techniques of recording, and characteristics of the normal EEG. *Am J EEG Technol* 1986;26:81–103.

Mizrahi EM. Electroencephalographic video monitoring in neonates, infants, and children. *J Child Neurol Suppl* 1994;9:s46–s56.

Mizrahi EM. Acute and chronic effects of seizures in the developing brain: Lessons from clinical experience. *Epilepsia* 1999;suppl 1:S42–S50.

Mizrahi EM. Neonatal seizures and neonatal epileptic syndromes. *Neurol Clin* 2001;19:427–463.

Mizrahi EM, Clancy RR. Neonatal seizures: early-onset seizure syndromes and their consequences for development. *Ment Retard Dev Disabil Res Rev* 2000;6:229–241.

Mizrahi EM, Kellaway P. Characterization and classification of neonatal seizures. *Neurology* 1987;37:1837–1844.

Mizrahi EM, Kellaway P. *Diagnosis and management of neonatal seizures.* Philadelphia: Lippincott-Raven, 1998:181.

Mizrahi EM, Pollack MA, Kellaway P. Neocortical death in infants: Behavioral, neurologic, and electroencephalographic characteristics. *Pediatr Neurol* 1985;1:302–305.

Mizrahi EM, Tharp BR. A characteristic EEG pattern in neonatal herpes simplex encephalitis. *Neurology* 1982;32:1215–1220.

Mizrahi EM, Watanabe K. Symptomatic neonatal seizures. In: Roger J, Bureau M, Dravet C, Genton P, Tassinari CA, Wolf P, eds. *Epileptic syndromes in infancy, childhood and adolescence,* 3rd ed. London: John Libbey & Co., 2002:15–31.

Monod D, Dreyfus-Brisac C, Ducas P, et al. L'EEG du nouveau-né à terme. Étude comparative chez le nouveau-né en présentation céphalique et en presentation de siège. *Rev Neurol* 1960;102:375–379.

Monod N, Pajot N. Le sommeil du nouveau-né et du prématuré, I: Analyse des études polygraphiques (mouvements oculaires, respiration et EEG chez le nouveau-né à terme). *Biol Neonat* 1965;8:281–307.

Monod N, Pajot N, Guidasci S. The neonatal EEG: Statistical studies and prognostic value in full-term and pre-term babies. *Electroencephalogr Clin Neurophysiol* 1972;32:529–544.

Navelet Y, D'Allest AM, Dehan M, Gabilan JC. A propos du syndrome des convulsions néonatales du cinquième jour. *Rev EEG Neurophysiol* 1981;11:390–396.

Nguyen T, Tich S, Vecchierini MF, et al. Effects of sufentanil on electroencephalogram in very and extremely preterm neonates. *Pediatrics* 2003;111:123–128.

Novotny EJ Jr, Tharp BR, Coen RW, et al. Positive rolandic sharp waves in the EEG of the premature infant. *Neurology* 1987;37:1481–1486.

O'Brien MJ, Lems YL, Prechtl HFR. Transient flattenings in the EEG of newborns: A benign variation. *Electroencephalogr Clin Neurophysiol* 1987;67:16–26.

Ohtahara S. Clinico-electrical delineation of epileptic encephalopathies in childhood. *Asian Med J* 1978;21:499–509.

Ohtahara S, Ohtsuka Y, Yamatogi Y, et al. Early-infantile epileptic encephalopathy with suppression-bursts. In: Roger J, Bureau M, Dravet C, et al., eds. *Epileptic syndromes in infancy, childhood, and adolescence,* 2nd ed. London: John Libbey, 1992:25–34.

Oliveira AJ, Nunes ML, Haertel LM, et al. Duration of rhythmic EEG patterns in neonates: new evidence for clinical and prognostic significance of brief rhythmic discharges. *Clin Neurophysiol.* 2000;111:1646–1653.

Ortibus EL, Sum JM, Hahn JS. Predictive value of EEG for outcome and epilepsy following neonatal seizures. *Electroencephalogr Clin Neurophysiol* 1996;98:175–185.

Painter MJ, Scher MS, Stein AD, et al. Phenobarbital compared with phenytoin for the treatment of neonatal seizures. *N Engl J Med* 1999;341:485–489.

Perlman JM, Volpe JJ. Seizures in the preterm infant: effects on cerebral blood flow velocity, intracranial pressure, and arterial blood pressure. *J Pediatr* 1983;102:288–293.

Pezzani C, Radvanyi-Bouvet MF, Relier JP, et al. Neonatal electroencephalography during the first twenty-four hours of life in full-term newborn infants. *Neuropediatrics* 1986;17:11–18.

Pinto LC, Giliberti P. Neonatal seizures: background EEG activity and the electroclinical correlation in full-term neonates with hypoxic-ischemic encephalopathy: Analysis by computer-synchronized long-term polygraphic video-EEG monitoring. *Epileptic Disord* 2001;3:125–132.

Plouin P. Benign idiopathic neonatal convulsions. In: Roger J, Bureau M, Dravet CH, Dreifuss FE, Perret A, Wolf P, eds. *Epileptic syndromes in infancy, childhood and adolescence,* 2nd ed. London: John Libbey & Co., 1992:3–11.

Plouin P. [Value of video electroencephalography in neonatology]. *Arch Pediatr* 2000;suppl 2:332s–333s.

Plouin P, Anderson VE. Epileptic syndromes in neonates In: Roger J, Bureau M, Dravet C, Genton P, Tassinari CA, Wolf P, eds. *Epileptic syndromes in infancy, childhood and adolescence,* 3rd ed. London: John Libbey & Co., 2002:3–13.

Rennie JM. Neonatal seizures. *Eur J Pediatr* 1997;156:83–87.

Rose AL, Lombroso CT. Neonatal seizure states. *Pediatrics* 1970;45:404–425.

Sainte-Anne-Dargassies S, Berthault F, Dreyfus-Brisac C, et al. La convulsion du tout jeune nourrisson; aspects électroencéphalographiques du probleme. *Presse Med* 1953;46:965–966.

Saunders MG. Artifacts: Activity of noncerebral origin in the EEG. In: Klass DW, Daly DD, eds. *Current practice of clinical electroencephalography,* 1st ed. New York: Raven Press, 1979:37–67.

Scher MS. Physiological artifacts in neonatal electroencephalography: The importance of technical comments. *Am J EEG Technol* 1985;25:257–277.

Scher MS. Seizures in the newborn infant: Diagnosis, treatment, and outcome. *Clin Perinatol* 1997;24:735–772.

Scher MS. Controversies regarding neonatal seizure recognition. *Epileptic Disord* 2002;4:139–158.

Scher MS, Aso K, Beggarly ME, et al. Electrographic seizures in preterm and full-term neonates: Clinical correlates, associated brain lesions, and risk for neurologic sequelae. *Pediatrics* 1993;91:128–134.

Scher MS, Beggarly M. Clinical significance of focal periodic discharges in neonates. *J Child Neurol* 1989;4:175–185.

Schulte FJ. Neonatal EEG and brain maturation: Facts and fallacies [Letter]. *Dev Med Child Neurol* 1970;12:396–399.

Selton D, Andre M. Prognosis of hypoxic-ischaemic encephalopathy in full-term newborns: Value of neonatal electroencephalography. *Neuropediatrics* 1997;28:276–280.

Selton D, Andre M, Hascoët JM. Normal EEG in very premature infants: reference criteria. *Clin Neurophysiol* 2000;111:2116–2124.

Sperber EF, Haas KZ, Stanton PK, Moshe SL. Resistance of the immature hippocampus to seizure-induced synaptic reorganization. *Brain Res Dev Brain Res* 1991;60:88–93.

Stafstrom CE, Holmes GL. Effects of uncontrolled seizures: Neural changes in animal models. *Adv Exp Med Biol* 2002;497:171–194.

Stafstrom CE, Thompson JL, Holmes GL. Kainic acid seizures in the developing brain: status epilepticus and spontaneous recurrent seizures. *Brain Res Dev Brain Res* 1992;65:227–236.

Swann JW. Recent experimental studies of the effects of seizures on brain development. *Prog Brain Res* 2002;135:391–393.

Swann JW, Hablitz JJ. Cellular abnormalities and synaptic plasticity in seizure disorders of the immature nervous system. *Ment Retard Dev Disabil Res Rev* 2000;6:258–267.

Takeuchi T, Watanabe K. The EEG evolution and neurological prognosis of neonates with perinatal hypoxia. *Brain Dev* 1989;11:115–120.

Tharp BR. Electrophysiological brain maturation in premature infants: An historical perspective. *J Clin Neurophysiol* 1990;7:302–314.

Tharp BR. Neonatal seizures and syndromes. *Epilepsia* 2002;suppl 3:2–10.

Tharp BR, Cukier F, Monod N. The prognostic value of the electroencephalogram in premature infants. *Electroencephalogr Clin Neurophysiol* 1981;51:219–236.

Tharp BR, Scher MS, Clancy RR. Serial EEGs in normal and abnormal infants with birth weights less than 1200 grams: A prospective study with long term follow-up. *Neuropediatrics* 1989;20:64–72.

Thurber SJ, Mikati MA, Stafstrom CE, Jensen FE, Holmes GL. Quisqualic acid-induced seizures during development: a behavioral and EEG study. *Epilepsia* 1994;35:868–875.

Torres F, Anderson C. The normal EEG of the human newborn. *J Clin Neurophysiol* 1985;2:89–103.

Torres F, Blaw ME. Longitudinal EEG-clinical correlations in children from birth to 4 years of age. *Pediatrics* 1968;41:945–954.

Velisek L, Moshe SL. Effects of brief seizures during development. *Prog Brain Res* 2002;135:355–364.

Villeneuve N, Ben-Ari Y, Holmes GL, et al. Neonatal seizures induced persistent changes in intrinsic properties of CA1 rat hippocampal cells. *Ann Neurol* 2000;47:729–738.

Volpe J. Neonatal seizures. *N Engl J Med* 1973;289:413–415.

Watanabe K, Iwase K, and Hara K. Development of slow-wave sleep in low birth weight infants. *Dev Med Child Neurol* 1974;16:23–31.

Watanabe K, Hara K, Miyazaki S, et al. Electroclinical studies of seizures in the newborn. *Folia Psychiatry Neurol Jpn* 1977;31:383–392.

Watanabe K, Hara K, Miyazaki S, Hakamada S, Kuroyanagi M. Apneic seizures in the newborn. *Am J Dis Child* 1982;136:980–984.

Watanabe K, Hayakawa F, Okumura A. Neonatal EEG: A powerful tool in the assessment of brain damage in preterm infants. *Brain Dev* 1999;21:361–372.

Watanabe K, Iwase K. Spindle-like fast rhythm in the EEGs of low birth weight infants. *Dev Med Child Neurol* 1972;14:373–381.

Werner SS, Stockard JE, Bickford RG. *Atlas of neonatal electroencephalography.* New York: Raven Press, 1977:401.

Willis J, Gould JB. Periodic alpha seizures with apnea in a newborn. *Develop Med Child Neurol* 1980;22:214–222.

Yakovlev PI. Pathoarchitectonic studies of cerebral malformations, III: Arhinencephalies (holotelencephalies). *J Neuropathol Exp Neurol* 1959;18:22–25.

Young GB, da Silva OP. Effects of morphine on the electroencephalograms of neonates: A prospective, observational study. *Clin Neurophysiol* 2000;111:1955–1960.

Zeinstra E, Fock JM, Begeer JH, et al. The prognostic value of serial EEG recordings following acute neonatal asphyxia in full-term infants. *Eur J Paediatr Neurol* 2001;5:155–160.

# Subject Index